Digital Diseases

Gökmen H. Karadağ (ed.)

Digital Diseases

PETER LANG

Bibliographic Information published by the Deutsche Nationalbibliothek
The Deutsche Nationalbibliothek lists this publication in the Deutsche Nationalbibliografie; detailed bibliographic data is available online at http://dnb.d-nb.de.

Library of Congress Cataloging-in-Publication Data
A CIP catalog record for this book has been applied for at the Library of Congress.

Printed by CPI books GmbH, Leck

@kentoh/shutterstock.com

ISBN 978-3-631-80553-4 (Print)
E-ISBN 978-3-631-81165-8 (E-PDF)
E-ISBN 978-3-631-81166-5 (EPUB)
E-ISBN 978-3-631-81167-2 (MOBI)
DOI 10.3726/b16574

Peter Lang – Berlin · Bern · Bruxelles · New York · Oxford · Warszawa · Wien

This publication has been peer reviewed.

www.peterlang.com

Preface

Since the beginning of this century, humanity has been struggling to stay afloat in a digital communication pool into which it was, so to speak, pushed suddenly. It has swallowed plenty of water while trying to take an occasional breath. The English language word "immersion", which is used a few times in this book, describes this recent stage quite well. "Immersion", meaning "total submerging" or "dipping entirely" can have good or bad connotations. A mere 15–20 years ago we could hardly dare to stick our toes into this water, now we are in it up to our throats. We are on the one hand scared of being drowned in it while at the same time elated by the fact it lifts us up. What is going on: Are we drowning or taking off to fly?

We have entered a new age: no doubt about it! This is so, first and foremost, because of the reality of digital communications which surround us completely, leaving no corner of our lives untouched. It is the major determinant of this age. Hence, the question "Hey, wait a minute, what is going on?" has to be the paramount question of not only philosophy and literature, but also medicine and social sciences.

The question concerning what the media did to us always remained at the top of my agenda as a communication researcher. (As a practitioner, my uppermost question was what we could do with the communication media.) Starting graduate study on mass communications in 1968, I was struck by the Marshall McLuhan phenomenon. The Canadian professor of literature had been turned into a pop-culture icon. His aphorisms such as "The medium is the message" had gone viral, using today's jargon. Everybody was talking about it.

According to McLuhan, when the dominant medium of communication changed, so did the sense ratios of the users, and when this change was internalized, it affected all perceptual processes. For instance, the transition from oral culture where the sense of hearing is dominant to written culture where the sense of seeing is dominant had given rise to the emergence of a brand new kind of human being: The "individual"! This was the real effect, insisted McLuhan. The real effect was hidden in this message. There was no digital media at that time, but supremacy of television was complete. McLuhan argued that this new development putting an end to the reign of the written word pushed humanity into a new phase where tribal structures based on "participation" and "sharing" came into being. Humanity was on the threshold of a new stage similar to the early years of the printing press. Thanks to the performance of the electronic technology operating at the speed of light, the speed of physical transportation had become less important, leading to new notions of space and time, making instancy a global reality. And what about the new digital media? What would McLuhan have said about them?

In my opinion, McLuhan who underlined the importance of evolution and change in cognitive information handling processes in a holistic approach would have gone beyond looking at the findings used in the articles brought together here as personal abnormalities and health disorders and delve into the historical background of such phenomena. Undoubtedly, other "extreme" users of the previous media were diagnosed as "sick" and, for instance, labeled as "bookworms" or "TV addicts". Such users are naturally worthy of attention. But what is really important is not the extreme users who are considered "sick," but the great majority who seem to be using the new technology ever more.

I would agree with him no matter how striking the examples of personal disorders we encounter in these pages. I think that is where the greater question resides. We have to admit that many of us also manifest many of the "symptoms" of "sicknesses" mentioned under a variety of names. Cafes are full of "lovers" who would look at the telephone screens in their hands rather than into each other's eyes. The last thing we do before going to bed is also the first thing we do when we wake up: Looking at that screen. Our entire lives have undergone a fundamental change whether we are aware of it or not.

Consequently, the illnesses we suffer from have also changed. This is so, no matter where you go around the globe. Despite the fact that the search for a new equilibrium among various media has yet to reach its final stage, it is certainly possible to say that there has evolved a new "normal" according to which the human individual is defined as someone who is in a state of constant digital communication. We know that not only today, but also tomorrow belongs to digital technology. Again, therein lies the big question: Leaving those who appear "sick" or "addicted" aside, what is happening to the majority presumed to be healthy? What is happening to them socially, culturally, and civilizationally?

I do hope colleagues who have demonstrated the courage to confront this big question by focusing on individual uses at the micro-level will now move up to the macro-level by initiating new studies. Further, I also hope the following are among the questions they ask: Can democracy survive in societies dominated by digital media? Or, could such media be making not only certain individuals, but also institutions sick? Can we then say that the whole world suffers from some form of the digital maladies described in this book?

Haluk Şahin, Professor Emeritus.

Table of Contents

Introduction

Digital development not only marked today's world in terms of technology, but also transformed our social life into completely different forms, and it has moved our social practices to an utterly different media. While some of our practices in social life are moved into "social" media with different forms, how similar the word "social" in this definition to the "social" that we know, and we are used to is heavily discussed. Digital technology has created a digital representation of almost everything that is real, bringing the need for socialization to social media and the need for reality to virtual reality (VR) systems. Even possibility of VR and augmented reality (AR) will nearly become the competitor of tourism that we know is a striking example in terms of the extent of digitalization. Whereas a copy spreads over everywhere and it replaces the real, like Baudrillard pointed out, individuals are exposed to increasingly effect of uncertainty of boundaries between the real and the copy. In this sense, with the dizzier development of technology, one of the many aspects of the digital representation that penetrates all areas of life that is expected to be discovered is created by new technology's impacts on human health and behavior.

Some of these effects are due to VR, while the others are due to overuse of new media. The most striking example of technology using all the possibilities allowed by digital representation is tremendous improvements on VR applications. In the virtual world, where a techno copy of real environment, surrounding the living space of human is designed, digital representation replaces with real objects and subjects. This technology is regarded as successful as it isolates the individual from real environment and gives the individual the feeling of being in the virtual environment (VE), presented not in the real world. However, while VR applications penetrate more and more areas, and the use of highly practical display types, such as the head mounted display, is increasingly becoming easy to use, it is observed that VR has also triggered serious symptoms and negative effects on human health.

Another problem demonstrating the negative effects of the digital era on human health and behaviors is the excessive use of the new media. Together with the internet access increasingly becoming easy and cheap to use; people, with their smart phones, constantly use the virtual world to look at or watch something at home, work, in the streets, cafés, classes, toilets, in their beds, at dinner, and so on. Users follow the contents of the new media, especially of the social media with an incredible appetite, constantly moving their fingers through their mobile screens. This behavior which has almost turned into an addiction is not limited to mobile screens. Besides, users, as the phrase goes, have surrendered to the deep water of the internet with their laptops or desktops. People now keep their mobile screens or computers open even when they follow the traditional media, and they have adopted a new way of viewing as a reflex that is called multi-screen. Naturally, this excessive use causes some negative physical, social, and psychological results. These results have recently been dealt with under several terms, such as **technology addiction**, **internet addiction**, **game addiction**, **digital diseases**, **digital behavior disorders**, **pathological use of the internet;** and the number of those denominations for the digital era diseases are getting more and more day by day. At this point, it should be stated that even World Health Organization has classified excessive gaming as a health problem, that is to say, as a sickness.

The book tackles the abovementioned diseases, which the ones who live the digital representation of the reality, but not the reality itself have got. They are including, but not limited to the following: **"cybersickness"** resulted from exposure to the VEs, **"digital ecstasy"** for the ones who have isolated themselves from the real life and lost themselves in cyber spaces and fantasies, **"digital addiction"** for the ones having crossed the thin line between connectedness and addiction, **"digital game addiction"** that is significantly dangerous especially for our children, **"binge watching"** that reminds us of the famous Turkish poet Tevrik Fikret's well-known saying, which is "Eat, gentlemen eat; eat till you feel replete; eat till it makes you gag!" even though it was said for a different context; **"ego surfing"** which can be interpreted as the narcissism in the digital era, **"digital cynicism"** which makes us say that "Could some awkward people possibly be the modern representations of Diogenes?", and the effects of **frame rate change** on the user experience in VR… In this wide spectrum, both literature reviews and original studies regarding the diseases of the digital era are included in this book.

The first disease to be touched upon in the book is **cybersickness**. Complaints such as headache, nausea, vomiting, fatigue, sweating, drowsiness, eyestrain, blurred vision, and vertigo are the typical signs of motion sickness, which has a long history and different theories of its causes. However, all these complaints resulting from what people have been through in psychical realities have now turned into the problems they experience in simulators and VR as a result of the technological development. The studies on the health-related effects of VR applications that have become widespread in ranging from education to medicine, from industry to scientific researches, and from entertaining market to video game market are gradually increasing. The reason of this increase is that the abovementioned issue constitutes one of the most significant health and security problems that could affect the development of VR technology. As of the early 1990s, the reports documenting the psychophysiological effects and aftereffects of being in VEs, that is to say, cybersickness, have started to emerge. The ones who have developed the VE technology refer to a big research pool consisting of a lot of studies that have been conducted on "human factor in VEs" for years to get the information they need to understand which kinds of technical and design changes are required to satisfy users' needs without exposing them to negative effects. In this frame, there is a contribution to those studies by **And Algül, Deniz Yengin, Gökmen H. Karadağ, Ayten Övür** and **Tamer Bayrak** conducted in **Istanbul Aydin University VR Laboratory**. The aim of that study is, in accordance with uses and effects approach, to determine the negative effects resulted from the VR experience on the users, and to find out the factors related with those effects.

Ayten Övür, in her chapter entitled **"Digital Ecstasy as Escapist Fantasy Field in the Age of Technology"**, illuminates the digital ecstasy experienced by the human communities that have lost their interest and perception for the outside world, that have isolated themselves from the real life like sleepwalkers, and as a result, have dived into virtual lives and fantasies. Digital ecstasy refers to the condition of being ecstatic and numbed under the effects of simulations and fantasies emerged by developed technologies. Even though the reasons of digital ecstasy might show similarities with the effects of alcohol, drunkenness caused by alcohol gives one a sort of relieving feeling that might make one forget some desires. However, in digital ecstasy, forgetting of those desires cannot be mentioned; on the contrary, materializing them even virtually and achieving satisfaction is important. Ayten Övür, from the perspective of uses and gratifications approach, examines our relationship with social media that was initially used as a leisure time activity and to erase our boredom, but has gradually turned into a sort of duty that requires us to study hard and to overexert for it.

In their chapter called **"Digitally Connected and/or Addicted"**, **Deniz Yengin** and **Berkan Bayındır** question the difference between being connected and addicted in a world where over half of the world with the population of 7.6 billion use the internet; and more than half of 5 billion mobile users access to the internet via their smart phones; last but not the least nearly 360 thousand tweets are tweeted in 1 minute. Addiction is generally associated with uses and gratifications theory in communication studies. Media use gives individuals a chance to escape from the anxiety in the society they live in. The internet as a way of escaping from loneliness has reached a process during which it is firstly turned into a dependency, and gradually into an addiction. Yengin and Bayındır first give a summary of the literature on dependency and addiction, then assess the results of several studies conducted on the signs of addiction, and finally, enhance the terms "nomophobia"and "netlessphobia", which is the fear of lack of mobile phones and of the internet, respectively. Internet-addicted digital immigrants and natives generally demonstrate some characteristics like an intense interest in the internet, anxious behaviors in the environments without the internet, alienation from responsibilities, and exceeding of the duration of use. The situation has now reached to such a serious level that rehabilitation centers have been established in a number of countries. It can be clearly seen that human-made technology has turned humans into mechanical slaves who need treatment.

Didem Ataman Yengin, in her chapter entitled **"Digital Game Addiction"**, notes digital game addiction as a danger threatening our future, i.e., our children. Parents who cannot take their children to open-air and lead them to play outside because of the insufficient playgrounds as a result of unplanned urbanization, and because of increasing security issues reluctantly and desperately let their children spend time and play games online. However, those games are not innocent. Most parents state that their children cheer up during playtime; feel sad and start to cry when they lose the game; experience cramps out of excitement and adrenalin in their bodies; adopt highly serious manners, and "pretend" isolating themselves from the world outside during playtime. The most significant sociological problem is that children do not go out, talk to anyone, and engage in any communication even with their relatives living in the same house because they get the illusion that they have already been socialized in cyberspaces; also it harms the notion of family which is the cornerstone of society. One of the most significant psychological problems is that children who stick themselves on computer monitors in a room gradually become isolated, alienated, and adopt an excessive ambition and violence tendency, and demonstrate emotional insufficiencies, as well as the sense of incapability in parallel with the loss of success in real life. In this study, **Didem Ataman Yengin** assesses digital game addiction in the light of the responses to the questions addressed to 350 students consisting of 1st, 2nd, 3rd, and 4th grades in some primary schools in Istanbul who play a game called ROBLOX and 245 family members.

Nur Emine Koç, in her chapter titled **"Binge Watching"**, points out another danger waiting us together with the development of technology, which is "binge watching", used to refer to watching episodes of series one after another. Koç, with the purpose of revealing the underlying reasons of binge watching and the effects of it on watchers, has examined why the watchers prefer to watch the digital platform series they actively watch, which series are preferred by the watchers displaying binge watching behavior, and what are the permanent effects of that binge watching on those watchers. Addictive digital platform series whose numbers are gradually increasing isolate watchers from the real life, sometimes taking the whole day of the watchers. Binge watching, which could cause several health problems, such as heart disease, blood pressure disorders, obesity, and cancer as a result of excessive immobility has now become an issue in Turkey too. Considering the proliferation of digital platforms and the habits of the internet use, especially of the young population, it has been determined that the series and movies market will mostly maintain its existence on digital platforms, and that binge watching behavior will become widespread. On such a significant issue, Koç has conducted a focus group study through the individuals who watch the series on Netflix, Puhu TV, BluTV and dizimag5.co, which is a foreign series digital platform, and reached some striking results.

Özge Topçu, in her chapter called **"Online Narcissism"**, tackles ego surfing. As known, one of the terms that have become popular together with the proliferation of the internet use is the internet surfing. However, now that what is being searched on the internet has become the individual himself or herself, another problem called ego surfing comes into existence. Ego surfing is described as the behavior in which some of the people who are fond of technology constantly search for their own names on the internet and follow the updates regarding their lives, feel happy when they find any information or like for them, but discomfort otherwise. This study concentrates on the definition of online narcissism, how it has emerged, and how it can be dealt with. With a survey of 20 questions, it has been aimed to determine the users' internet addiction, their perception for the extent to which they are narcissist, and how often they search for their names.

Hakan Tan, in his chapter entitled **"Digital Cynicism"**, questions whether cynicism is also observed in digital space or not, based on behaviors and discourses of the individuals (actors) on some social media platforms they deal with. Does digital cynicism exist? Is digital cynicism a disorder that needs to be treated? What is normal, and what is abnormal? Is cynicism a dangerous philosophy for the society, or is it possible for it to have a positive function of stimulus for the society? Tan, in his study embracing these critical questions with nuances, discusses whether cynically fundamental behaviors and discourses are observed on some social media samples or not. Tan questions whether cynicism, a highly special term in terms of its philosophical history, is experienced as digital cynicism today. In this study, some samples that display cynical behaviors without possibly not acting with the awareness of cynicism, i.e., unconsciously display them are interpreted.

Tamer Bayrak and **And Algül**, in their chapter titled with **"Effects of Frame Rate in Virtual Reality"**, have examined the effects of frame rate factor on the users of VR. Some of the effects induced by VR are associated with the features of the provided VE. One of those features is frame rate. Bayrak and Algül have studied whether Frame per Second (FPS) change has any effects on the users during the use of head mounted displays or not, and what these effects are if it does. Through a suitable sampling with 50 people, the users experienced four different VR games with various levels of FPS change; the users' performance was observed during the play, and at the end of the play, they were asked questions in order to measure their experiences of use.

Digital sicknesses, digital diseases, or digital behavior disorders certainly spread to a lot wider spectrum than listed here. However, in this book, the scope has been limited to those abovementioned titles. As new studies are conducted on both the titles included and not included in this book, a better comprehension and more data on the new diseases of today's world called the internet era will emerge, and these studies will also guide us to find the ways to deal with those diseases and develop defense mechanisms against them.

Asst. Prof. Dr. Gökmen H. Karadağ

And Algül, Deniz Yengin, Gökmen H. Karadağ, Ayten Övür,
and Tamer Bayrak

Cybersickness

Abstract: Complaints such as headache, nausea, vomiting, fatigue, sweating, drowsiness, eyestrain, blurred vision, and vertigo are the typical signs of motion sickness, which has a long history and different theories of its causes. However, all these complaints resulting from what people have been through in psychical realities have now turned into the problems they experience in simulators and virtual reality (VR) as a result of the technological development. The studies on the health-related effects of the VR applications that have become widespread in ranging from education to medicine, from industry to scientific researches, and from entertaining market to video game market are gradually increasing. The reason of this increase is that the abovementioned issue constitutes one of the most significant health and security problems that could affect the development of VR technology. As of the early 1990s, the reports documenting the psychophysiological effects and aftereffects of being in VEs, that is to say, cybersickness, have started to emerge. The ones who have developed the VE technology refer to a big research pool consisting of a lot of studies that have been conducted on "human factor in VE's" for years to get the information they need to understand which kinds of technical and design changes are required to satisfy users' needs without exposing them to negative effects. As a contribution to those studies, the aim of this study is, in accordance with uses and effects approach, to determine the negative effects resulted from the VR experience on the users, and to find out the factors related with those effects.

Keywords: virtual reality, virtual environment, cybersickness, simulator sickness, motion sickness

Introduction

One of the most important health and safety issues that may influence the advancement of Virtual Environment (VE) technology is cybersickness. Cybersickness is a form of motion sickness that occurs as a result of exposure to VEs (Stanney et al., 1998: 341). Complaints like headache, vertigo, nausea, vomiting, and weakness are typical symptoms of motion sickness, which dates back to very old times and has various theories about its causes. With technological developments, such complaints resulting from what people go through in physical reality have also become the complaints of simulator and cyberspace users.

Information on how people act and orient themselves according to environmental reference frames is respectively called self-motion information and

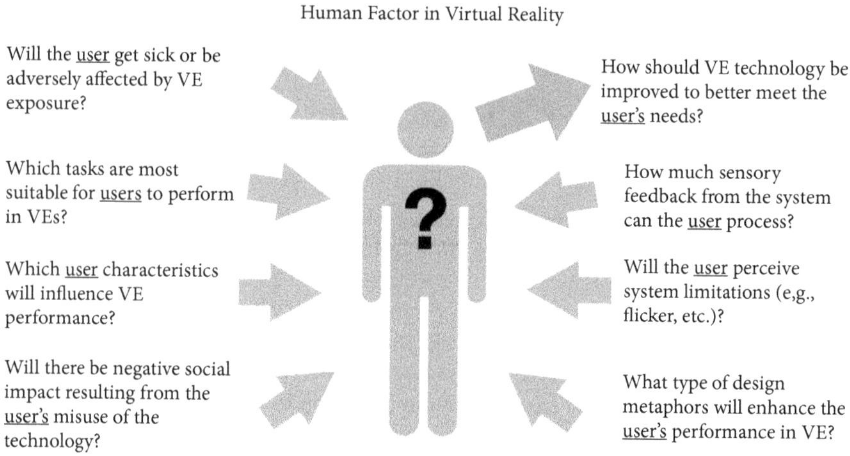

Fig. 1: Human Factor in Virtual Environments (Stanney et al., 1998: 328).

self-orientation information. Distortion of self-orientation and self-motion information may lead to postural disturbance and motion sickness (Duh et al., 2004: 142). Although the stimuli and triggering mechanisms for motion sickness, simulator sickness, and cybersickness are different, their symptoms overlap to a great extent. There has been a lot of research both on the causes, intensity, and incidence of symptoms, and on alleviating and eliminating adverse effects. Examining and questioning the interaction between man and virtual environment, these studies are of particular concern to the future of cyberspace sector. Here is the main question to be answered: In what way can one develop virtual environment technology to meet users' needs better? Other questions to be answered in order to illuminate this fundamental issue are shown in Fig. 1.

The developers of virtual environment technology benefit from the pool of studies on the human factor in VEs that have been carried out for years, and thanks to those studies, they acquire the relevant knowledge as to what changes in techniques and designs are required to meet users' needs without exposing them to adverse effects.

In the future, it is possible that virtual environment technology which is employed mainly in gaming industry at present is likely to replace communication devices we use today. In this context, the objective of our study is to illuminate negative effects of the use of cyberspace according to the uses and effects approach and to explore the relationship between these negative effects and factors.

Cybersickness

The term "cybersickness" was coined by McCauley and Sharkey to describe the motion-sickness-like symptoms associated with virtual environments. McCauley and Sharkey proposed this term to differentiate it from simulator sickness because they regarded simulator sickness as a subset of motion sickness suffered while surfing virtual environments (1992: 313). The term "simulator sickness" was coined to describe motion-sickness-like reactions observed in driving simulators and military flight simulators (Kolasinski, 1995: 2). The expression of "Virtual Reality Induced Symptoms and Effects" (VRISE) is also used instead of cybersickness (Cobb et al., 1999; Nichols et al., 2000; Sharples et al., 2008). Another term is "Synthetic Experience" proposed to describe experiences in virtual environments and simulators (Lawson et al., 2002).

As can be seen, "motion-sickness-like symptoms" is used in the definitions of both simulator sickness and cybersickness. The term "motion sickness" was proposed by Irwin in 1881 to provide a general designation for such similar syndromes as seasickness, train sickness, and the like (Graybiel, 1988: 44). At first, motion sickness was known to be caused only by the real motion on land, at sea, and in the air. However, later on, it was understood that synthetic experiences such as fixed- or moving-base simulators, VEs, teleoperators, augmented reality, and large-screen or 3D movies also cause motion sickness (Lawson, 2014: 532).

Data provided by the vestibular system play an important role in the formation of motion sickness. There are three semi-circular canals for detecting angular acceleration, and the utricle and saccule detect linear acceleration in the vestibular system in the inner ear (see Fig. 2). The three semi-circular canals correspond to each of the three dimensions in which human movement can take place (Gleitman, 1992; as cited in LaViola, 2000: 49). Data provided by the receptors detecting motion in three levels are combined with data from the eye, and all the information is interpreted in the central nervous system so that motor messages enabling the body to stand in balance are formed and the eyeball is moved (Büyükkurt et al., 2008: 109). The vestibular system is arguably one of the most ancient vertebrate sensory systems. Its evolution enabled vertebrates to detect and control their own motion in any environment (Higstein, 2004: 1). Motion sickness is a common consequence of vestibular disease. Virtually everyone is susceptible to some degree, provided the stimulus is appropriate and lasts long enough. (Oman, 1991: 362).

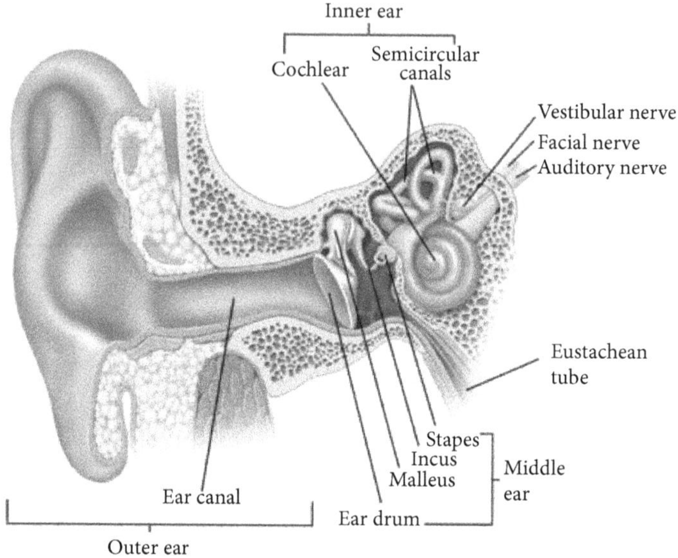

Fig. 2: An Illustration of Vestibular System (Lu, 2016: 15).

Originally, it was assumed that motion sickness can only be caused by motion. However, by 1970 some forms of motion sickness were recognized in which head and body motion is normal or even absent (Oman, 1998: 51). These forms of motion sickness were described first in simulators and then in cyberspace applications, and they were widely examined. Visual stimulation, not vestibular one, is on both in simulator sickness and in cybersickness. However, motion sickness can be triggered only by vestibular stimuli, even if visual factors play a role (LaViola, 2000: 47). The most commonly accepted causes of cybersickness are the sensory and perceptual mismatches that occur between the visual and vestibular systems. Cybersickness is an unintended psychophysiological response to exposure to the perceptual illusions of VEs (Barret, 2004; 4). Cybersickness has been described not just as polysymptomatic, but also as polygenic due to the diversity of both causative factors and symptoms (Kennedy et al., 1993; as cited in Barret, 2004: 38). Cybersickness, the result of unintended side effects of participation in VEs, is a complex problem that can reduce the effectiveness of VEs and cause potential health and safety problems (Barret, 2004: 37). Cybersickness poses a serious threat to the usability of VR systems (Stanney et al., 1998: 341).

Symptoms of Cybersickness and Assessment Questionnaires

There are common and different symptoms of motion sickness, simulator sickness, and cybersickness. Based on the frequency and severity of these symptoms, several assessment questionnaires have been developed for each sickness. In fact, both simulator sickness and VE sickness are forms of motion sickness. In other words, identifying and assessing symptoms started with motion sickness questionnaires. However, studies have shown that simulator sickness and VE sickness are triggered by such different factors in such different cases that it is necessary to assess them with a different questionnaire.

The most widely used questionnaire for the assessment of motion sickness is the Pensacola Diagnostic Index (PDI) (Graybiel et al., 1968; as cited in Gianaros et al., 2001: 1). The Motion Sickness Questionnaire (MSQ) is used to assess various forms of motion and visually induced sickness (Barret, 2004: 9). The Pensacola MSQ consists of a list of 25–30 symptoms. Participants give information on the presence and degree of severity of symptoms, which are converted to scores on a scale (Kennedy et al., 1993: 204). However, this index yields a single score that depends on the composite magnitude of the following symptoms: nausea, dizziness, headache, warmth, sweating, and drowsiness. Conversely, the fact that the quantitative feature of motion sickness is determined to be a multidimensional construct with several symptom components is regarded as a better alternative. In this approach, simulator sickness is examined in terms of the following dimensions: (1) oculomotor (eyestrain, difficulty focusing, blurred vision, and headache), (2) disorientation (dizziness and vertigo) and (3) nausea (nausea, stomach awareness, increased salivation, and burping) (Gianaros, 2001: 2).

After a series of factor analyses of a large database of results obtained by administering the Pensacola MSQ to pilots following simulator hops, Simulator Sickness Questionnaire (SSQ) was prepared (Barret, 2004: 9). The patterns of symptom presence and severity associated with Simulator Sickness are sufficiently different from those of motion sickness to justify the use of separate measuring systems (Kennedy et al., 1993: 219). Some of the symptoms in the MSQ are almost never reported under simulator exposure, or, if noted, are indicated at a level that fails to exceed a base level (Kennedy et al., 1993: 205). Because flight simulation technology involves stimulus conditions that produce visual distortion, and visual/motion transport delays and asynchronies that are ordinarily absent in environments that produce sea and air sickness (Kennedy et al., 1993: 204). Transport delay is the delay between the action and the corresponding rendering cues (Kemeny, 2014: 1). Thus, an SSQ shorter than the

Tab. 1: Symptoms in Motion Sickness Questionnaire (MSQ) and Simulator Sickness Questionnaire (SSQ) (Kennedy et al., 1993: 206)

MSQ Symptom	Retained for SSQ	Eliminated for SSQ
General discomfort	X	
Fatigue	X	
Boredom		X
Drowsiness		X
Headache	X	
Eyestrain	X	
Difficulty focusing	X	
Increased salivation	X	
Decreased salivation		X
Sweating	X	
Nausea	X	
Difficulty concentrating	X	
Depression		X
Fullness of head	X	
Blurred vision	X	
Dizziness (eyes open)	X	
Dizziness (eyes closed)	X	
Vertigo	X	
Visual flashbacks		X
Faintness		X
Awareness of breathing		X
Stomach awareness	X	
Decreased appetite		X
Increased appetite		X
Desire to move bowels		X
Confusion		X
Burping	X	
Vomiting		X

MSQ was developed. Tab. 1 indicates what symptoms in the MSQ are present and absent in the SSQ.

Cybersickness has both symptoms and dimensions in common with simulator sickness. As in simulator sickness, symptoms are divided into three groups: nausea, disorientation, and oculomotor effects (Barret, 2004: 37). With regard to how dominant these three groups are, differences between simulator sickness and VE sickness have been discovered. Stanney et al. listed the symptom groups for the two sicknesses according to their dominance as such: for simulator sickness, (1) oculomotor, (2) nausea, and (3) disorientation; for VE sickness, (1) disorientation, (2) nausea, and (3) oculomotor. Moreover, the total severity of VE sickness is found to be about three times greater than that of simulator sickness (Stanney et al., 1997: 1138). This is explained by the fact that VE systems provide a stronger or a fundamentally different stimulus than simulator systems (Stanney et al., 1997: 1140).

Theories on Cybersickness

For a long time, researchers have been looking into the similar and different symptoms and causes of motion sickness, simulator sickness, and cybersickness, and dealing with factor analyses. New theories on how sicknesses emerge were gradually added to the old ones, and some of these were thought to be conflicting. Thus, one can often encounter literature summarizing these three sicknesses (Barrett, 2004; Costello, 1997; Johnson, 2005; LaViola, 2000; Lawson, 2014; Nichols et al., 2000; Stanney, 2002). Although there are many suggestions about the causes of cybersickness, to date there are no definitive predictive theories; however, there are models in general (Stanney et al., 1998: 341).

Sensory Conflict Theory

The sensory conflict hypothesis was originally proposed by Claremont (1931) and has since been revised and extended by several authors (Oman, 1991: 364). It is also possible to call the theory sensory rearrangement. Motion sickness emerges when the rules which define the normal relationship between body movements and the resulting neural inflow to the central nervous system have been systematically changed, that is when people are exposed to conditions of sensory rearrangement (Reason, 1978: 827). Information supporting postural control and locomotion is provided by visual, vestibular auditory, and proprioceptive senses (McCauley and Sharkey, 1992: 312). In many simulators and VEs, the self-motion and self-orientation cues received by the vestibular receptors differ from those received by the visual receptors, and this cue conflict may be the basic cause for the sickness (Duh et al., 2004: 143).

When someone is in a stationary position, they can still get the impression of self-motion under certain conditions. This deceptive impression of self-motion is called vection. Vection can occur, for example, when someone is in a stationary vehicle while an adjacent vehicle begins to move. Vection can also be produced with wide field-of-view displays (the same displays that are used in virtual environments) of optical flow patterns that are characteristic of self-motion (Harwood and Foley, 1987; as cited in LaViola, 2000: 49). In a fixed-base simulator, the visual system senses motion while the vestibular system senses no motion. Thus, according to the cue conflict theory, a conflict emerges. In a moving-base simulator, the visual stimuli experienced may not correspond exactly to the motion which the vestibular system registers. Thus, a conflict can still result (Kolasinski, 1995: 7).

Even though the sensory conflict theory explains the motion sickness to some extent, it is inadequate. The sensory conflict theory claims that a cue conflict can cause cybersickness, but it does not provide an explanation for why such a conflict could make someone sick (LaViola, 2000: 51; Oman, 1998: 52). What is more, it does not account for why some individuals get sick and why others do not when given a set of identical stimuli (LaViola, 2000: 51).

Postural Instability Theory

Criticizing the sensory conflict theory, Riccio and Stoffregen proposed the postural instability theory to explain the sickness. In their opinion, the fact that vestibular and visual systems produce different data is not a conflict, but a case of complementary information, and the conflict theory does not explain why this case does not cause the sickness in many occasions (Riccio and Stoffregen, 1991: 197). According to Riccio and Stoffregen's theory, prolonged postural instability is the cause of motion sickness (1991: 231). According to the postural instability theory, one of the primary behavioural goals in humans is to maintain postural stability, which is defined as the state in which uncontrolled movements of the perception and action systems are minimized (Riccio and Stoffregen, 1991: 199). Whenever the environment changes in an abrupt or significant way, in many cases, postural control will be lost especially if the control strategies are not available due to lack of experience (LaViola, 2000: 51). Since in many VEs there are optically specified accelerations and rotations that are unrelated to the constraints on control of the body, postural control strategies for gaining postural stability will not work (LaViola, 2000: 52).

Toxin Theory (or Poison Theory)

A lesser known theory, the poison theory, claims that the cause of cybersickness is based on a maladaptive process which originally used to help the body get rid of toxic substances (LaViola, 2000: 54). Motion sickness is triggered by difficulties which arise in the programming of movements of the eyes or head when the relations between the spatial frameworks defined by the visual, vestibular, or proprioceptive inputs are repeatedly and unpredictably perturbed. Stating that such perturbations may be produced by certain types of motion, or by disturbances in sensory input or motor control produced by ingested toxins, Treisman thinks that the last would be the important cause in nature, the main function of the emesis being to rid the individual of ingested neurotoxins. Its occurrence in response to motion would be an accidental by-product of this system (Treisman, 1977: 493).

There are pros and cons of the three theories explaining how and why motion sickness and its versions —simulator and cyberspace sicknesses— occur. All three theories present valid arguments for the cause of cybersickness, yet in each theory an example for when the theory does not hold can be found. Moreover, they do not have a firm grasp for why one individual gets sick while another does not in identical conditions (LaViola, 2000: 54). At the most general level, there is still no consensus as to the reason why motion sickness should occur. Equally the reasons for the great individual differences in motion sickness susceptibility are still only poorly understood (Golding, 2006: 73). When great differences between users, the variety of equipment in virtual environments, and the diverse tasks in the applications in VEs demanded to be completed by users are considered, it is almost impossible to precisely predict the effect of a task in a specific system application upon a user (Oman, 1991: 363).

Factors Affecting Cybersickness

Many studies carried out so far are about which factors affect motion-sickness-like symptoms in simulators and virtual environments. As a result, positive and negative relations between the factors explored and the sickness have been found. In some studies, however, no meaningful relation has been found. As can be seen in Tab. 2, Kolasinski lists potential factors associated with simulator sickness in virtual environments. There are individual factors, simulator factors (regarding the nature of virtual environments), and task factors (regarding what is done in the simulator in virtual environments).

There is a wide source of literature on the factors affecting the sickness resulting from the use of cyberspace. Many studies have yielded findings as to whether individual factors, cyberspace, and VE factors and task factors lead to the sickness, how severe the sickness is if those factors cause the sickness, what symptoms they trigger, and to what extent they trigger those symptoms. Most of the studies were carried out with similar methods. In these studies,

Tab. 2: Potential Factors Associated with Simulator Sickness in Virtual Environments (Kolasinski, 1995: 48)

Individual	Simulator	Task
• Age • Concentration level • Ethnicity • Experience with real-world task • Experience with simulator (adaptation)	• Binocular viewing • Calibration • Color • Contrast • Field of view (FOV) • Flicker	• Altitude above terrain • Degree of control • Duration • Global Visual Flow • Head movements • Luminance level
• Flicker fusion frequency threshold	• Inter-pupillary distance	• Method of movement
• Gender • Illness and personal characteristics • Mental rotation ability	• Motion platform • Phosphor lag • Position-tracking error	• Rate of linear or rotational acceleration • Self-movement speed
• Perceptual style	• Refresh rate	• Sitting vs. standing • Type of application
• Postural stability	• Resolution • Scene content • Time lag (Transport delay) • Update rate (frame rate)	• Unusual maneuvers • Vection

various VE applications were performed, and the presence and severity of the symptoms which were listed by the participants, many of which were immersed in the VE with head mounted displays, were measured. In some studies, however, cybersickness was not measured with subjective accounts, but with objective methods (in addition to subjective accounts). In other words, factors such as participants' pulse, heartbeat, brain waves, body and head movements, and eye tracking were checked.

Findings of Previous Studies on Cybersickness

As for the data on the rate of the experimental sample reporting sickness symptoms, Regan and Price (1993a and 1993b) found that 42 % of the total sample reported sickness during immersion, and 61 % reported sickness symptoms during or post immersion. Kolasinski (1996) found 30 % of the experimental sample experienced sickness (as cited in Nichols et al., 2000: 9). In the studies of Nichols et al., 70 % reported an increase in symptoms from pre-post

VE exposure (Nichols et al., 2000: iv). In the studies of Lawson et al., at least 60 % of the VE users reported negative symptoms in their first experience. At least 5 % of the whole users could not stand the use of the VE for a long time (Lawson et al., 2002: 596). In the study of Lampton et al., some users, between 4 % and 16 %, experienced discomfort to the extent that they terminated their participation (Lampton et al., 1994: 1154).

There are some studies on physiological changes associated with the sickness triggered by cyberspace. Calvert and Tan found that there is an increase in the heartbeat of subjects who performed some tasks and played cyberspace games, just as the scholars expected (1994: 135). Strickland and Cartier (1997) found that changes in EEG occurred post VR use, and Ramsey (1999) found that changes in salivary cortisol and heart rate occurred post VE use (as cited in Nichols et al., 2000: 9–10).

The relation between symptoms and various factors was also questioned:

Age Factor

According to Reason and Brand (1975), tendency to experience motion sickness is seen most between the ages of 2 and 12. After the age of 12, this tendency lessens, and it is barely seen after the age of 50 (as cited in Kolasinski, 1995: 17–18). However, the study by Brooks et al (2010) showed that people who are older than 50 years old are more likely to experience virtual reality sickness compared to younger adults (as cited in Lu, 2016: 14). Park et al. found higher symptom incidence for older drivers (Park et al., 2006: 2702). Braithwaite and Braithwaite (1990) found no relationship between age and reported SS. According to the study by Warner et al. (1993), the rate of those who could not complete the simulation is 37,5 % in the older group, and 6,25 % in the younger one; however, among those who completed the flight, there was no significant difference in discomfort ratings between the younger and older groups (as cited in Johnson, 2005: 39).

Gender Factor

Kennedy and Frank (1983) state that women might be more likely to experience motion sickness because they have a wider field of view than men (as cited in Kolasinski, 1995: 20). In the study by Park et al., no gender differences were found within the dropout group but in the non-dropout group women were found to be more likely to experience motion sickness resulting from the use of VEs (Park et al., 2006: 2702). In Lu's study, the female group have shown a higher level of symptom severeness compared to the male group, especially in stomach awareness (Lu, 2016: 40). Koslucher et al. observed in field studies that motion sickness is more common among women than among men; however, they explain the fact that this difference is not reflected enough in laboratory research with the usage of rotational motion stimuli. In their studies, where they used linear visual oscillation, they found that sickness occurrence in women is 38 %, and it is 9 % in men (Koslucher et al., 2015: 787). In the two experiments by Munafo et al., where they used Oculus Rift helmet-mounted display, they observed that motion sickness in women is more common (Munafo et al., 2017: 889).

Sickness and Individual Characteristics Factor

It is claimed that there is some connection between the tendency towards simulator sickness and many forms of sicknesses. Kennedy et al. (1987) recommended that those who do not feel that they are in normal health condition should not be exposed to simulator. Moreover, Biocca (1992) suggested that there might be a relationship between the tendency towards the sickness and individual characteristics such as neuroticism, anxiety, arousal, and introversion (as cited in Kolasinski, 1995: 20). In the study by Nichols et al., specific examination of a small number of participants with diagnosed classic migraine with aura indicated more adverse symptoms (Nichols et al., 2000: iv). In Lu's study, the people who have had previous motion sickness experiences tend to suffer a bit more from VR sickness. However, the differences between the two groups with different previous motion sickness experiences were insignificant according to the statistical calculation (Lu, 2016: 40). In the study by Lampton et al. (1995), SSQ points of the participants who reported previous motion sickness experiences were significantly high (as cited in Johnson, 2005: 42).

Real-Life and Simulator Experience Factor

According to several studies, there is a negative relationship between the sickness and real-life and simulator experience. However, not all findings are coherent in literature (Kolasinski, 1995: 18–19). Kennedy et al. (2000), who used the data collected from the 938 military flight simulations, demonstrated that symptoms tend to be less severe after a few repeated immersions (as cited in Bouchard et al., 2007: 117). In the study by Lampton et al., the points of the civilians in the motion sickness questionnaire were much higher than those of the navy pilots (Lampton et al., 1994: 1154–1156). Stoffregen et al. found that during virtual driving, drivers became motion sick more rapidly than non-drivers, but the incidence and severity of motion sickness did not differ as a function of driving experience (Stoffregen et al., 2017).

Screen Type Factor (Binocular Vision Factor)

There are also some studies regarding the connection between the sickness and VR system display type. Nichols et al. found that some participants do experience sickness symptoms as a result of viewing VEs on desktop, standard projection screen and Reality Theatre displays, but these symptoms are not as prevalent or severe as Head Mounted Display (HMD) viewing (Nichols et al., 2000: iv). Sharples et al. found that symptoms are triggered most by helmet-mounted display usage (Sharples et al., 2008: 68).

Field of View Factor

Both wide and narrow fields of view have been suggested to lead to motion sickness. Lestienne et al (1977) found that subjects who viewed a wide field of view (FOV) experienced intense sensations of motion sickness (as cited in Stanney et al., 1998: 341). Lin et al. found that with an increased FOV, participants got higher points in the SSQ (Lin et al., 2002: 169). Duh et al. claimed that an increased FOV leads to balance disorder, and this disorder is connected with the simulator sickness (Duh et al., 2002: 330). Nichols et al. stated that no consistent relationship between sickness and postural stability has been identified (Nichols et al., 2000: 10). Anderson and Braunstein (1985) emphasized that when the FOV is restricted, nausea occurs (as cited in Stanney et al., 1998: 341).

Duration of Exposure to VE Factor

Various studies have found a positive relationship between the presence and severity of symptoms and the duration of the exposure to VEs. According to Lampton et al., the duration of the exposure to VE appears to be a major determinant of symptom severity. Thus, the longer the exposure, the more severe the symptoms (Lampton et al., 1994: 1157). Howarth and Finch (1999) assessed nausea symptoms every minute with 14 civilians immersed for 20 minutes in a virtual environment. They found a progressive increase of symptoms over time. Kennedy et al. (2000) pointed out that more lengthy immersions trigger gradually increasing side effects (as cited in Bouchard et al., 2007: 117).

Before the presentation of findings, it is necessary to mention the theory upon which the study is based. The approach of uses and effects is derived from resorting to both effect studies and the approach of uses and gratifications. In this context, the model of uses and effects emphasizes the synthesis of paradigms of pleasure and effect (Dağtaş, 1994: 125–129; Tekinalp and Uzun, 2009: 119; Uzun, 2013: 97). According to uses and effects model, the type of the mass media content used, how much, and how it is used play a significant role to estimate the results of that content usage. Certain contents tend to demonstrate certain effects. Apart from that, the type of usage of mass media itself causes certain effects (Uzun, 2013:97). As for the symptoms induced by virtual reality, the determinants are personal factors, the features of the virtual environment used, and duration of exposure to the virtual environment, together with the content of the virtual environment; i.e., the qualities of the tasks performed by the users of virtual environment within that environment. Within the scope of our study, the effects of the use of VR glasses are explored, and its impacts on communication processes are predicted.

Findings

In this study on the symptoms induces by virtual reality, literature research was initially done relating to Motion Sickness, Simulator Sickness, and Virtual Reality Sickness. Laboratory possibilities were evaluated regarding how to detect the effects that were detected within the literature research. It was detected that participants of the research may experience games in four game genres under four different categories (Eagle Flight, Robots Rescue, Drive Club, Until Dawn), using three different virtual reality devices (using console, using move controllers, and only using the headset).

The genre of the first game, Eagle Flight, is action and it appeals to people at the age of 7 and above. In this game similar to "First Person Shooter", the participant wanders around the city using head motions from the eagle's perspective. Wandering around the city, the participant must find the eagle's nest and manoeuvre across the different parts of the city using head motions.

The second game, Robots Rescue, is an action game and appeals to people at the age of 3 and above. In this game played in the "Role Playing" way, the participant tries to save the other robots similar to himself or herself, collect the golds and run away from the monsters, driving one of the main character robots in the game (making it walk, jump, or walking on a rope).

The third game, Drive Club, is an action game and appeals to people at the age of 3 and above. In the game played in the "First Person Shooter" way, the participant races with the other cars in the track and tries to finish three rounds as soon as possible.

The fourth game, Until Dawn, is a horror game and appeals to people at the age of 18 and above. In the game, played in the "First Person Shooter" way, the participant must kill the zombies while moving towards the tunnel in the game place and gain points for shooting several stimuli in a certain time.

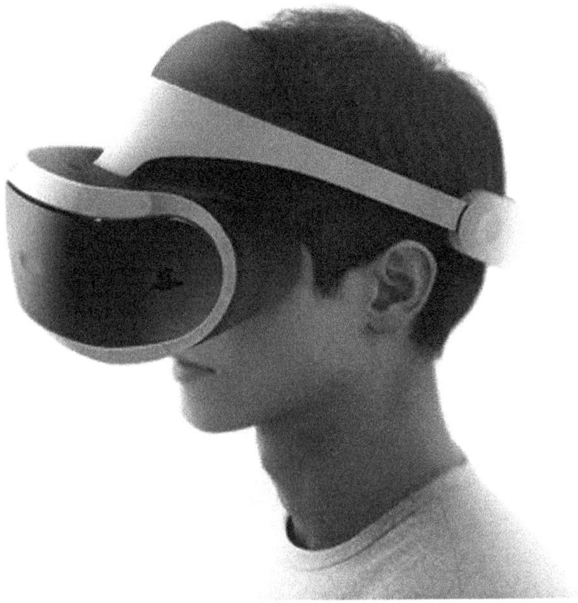

Fig. 3: Example of a Virtual Reality Headset. Eagle Flight Game Equipment (Smith, 2019).

The study was performed under doctor supervision in order to prevent unsolicited situations through the scope of the research period, meaning the period where participants experience the virtual reality headset. Attention was paid about whether participants of the research have a disease or not. Participants were allowed in the virtual reality laboratory (game zone) on an individual basis in order to prevent them from affecting each other, and they were warned regarding not talking about the experience with their friends.

In the context of usage and effects approach, the survey study was made with a 50-person focus group between the dates of 26 December 2017 and 20 March 2018, in order to reveal what are the negative effects that occur due to virtual reality usage experience and what demographic characteristics and/or factors these negative effects are related to. Participants were initially asked to fill out a 36-question survey consisting of demographic information. After the survey, participants were asked to experience four different games while standing up.

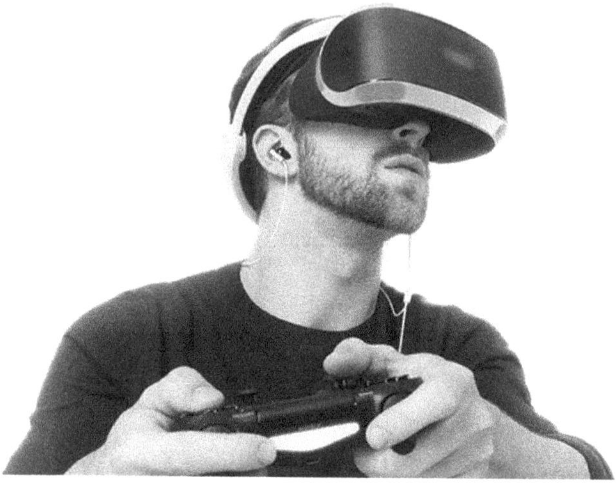

Fig. 4: Example of a Console Robots Game and Drive Club Game Equipment (The Nirvanist, 2016).

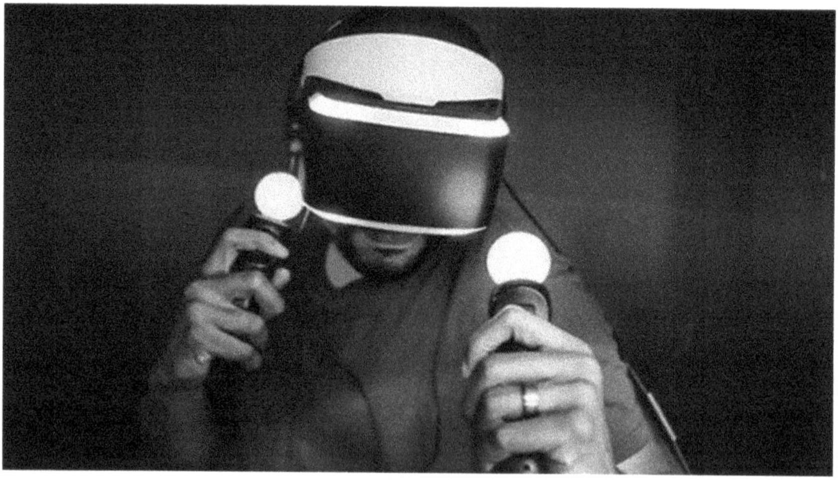

Fig. 5: Move Controllers. Until Dawn Game Equipment (Torre, 2014).

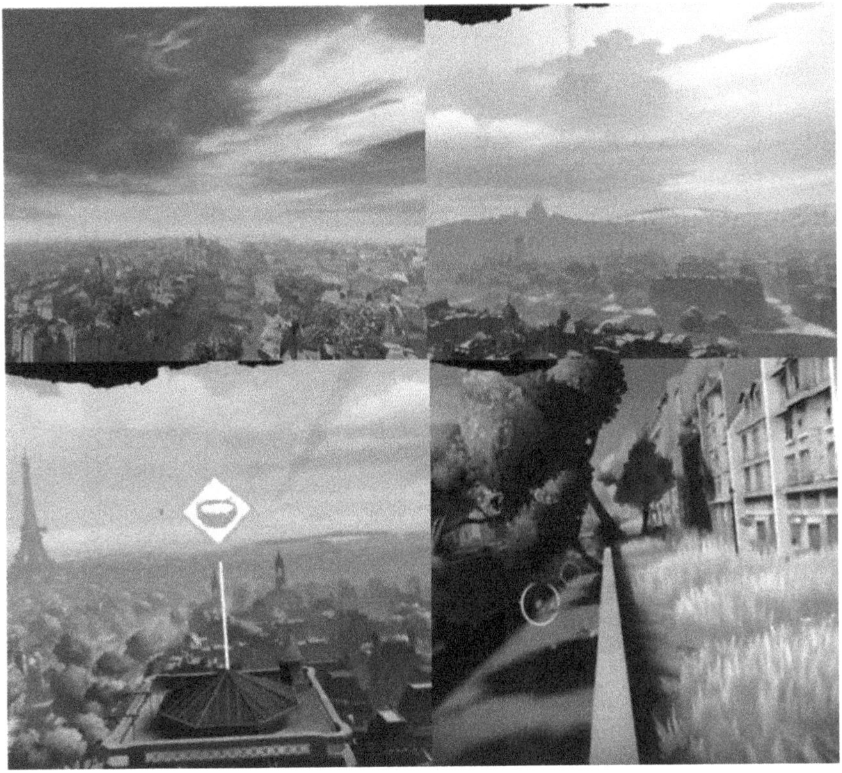

Fig. 6: Images from Eagle Flight (Eagle Flight, n.d.).

Experiences of each user in four different game genres were recorded. Participants were informed before the experience about what type of research they will be contributing to and what they are expected to do; and a letter of consent was signed that they participated in the research on their own free wills. Following the virtual reality headset experience, participants were asked to fill out a 52-question survey about whether they feel the negative effects or not.
Research question: "In the context of uses and effect approach, what are the negative effects of using a virtual reality tool and what demographic characteristics and factors are these negative effects related to?"

In this context, the research hypotheses are as follows:

Hypothesis 1: Virtual reality headsets have negative effects on users.

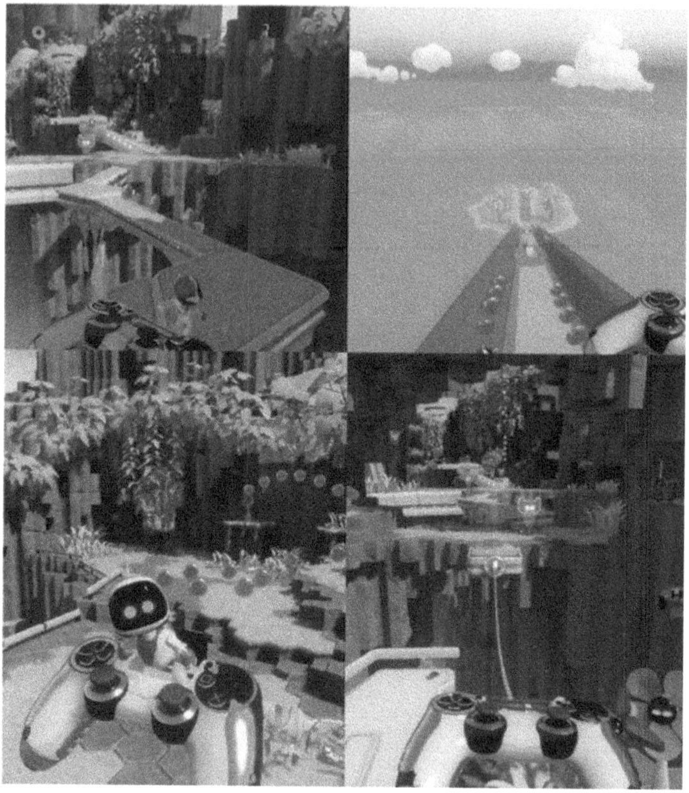

Fig. 7: Images from Robots Rescue (The VR Playroom, n.d.).

Hypothesis 2: As part of the digital gaming experience, virtual reality headsets are not yet widely used.

Hypothesis 3: Gamer experience formed as a result of the duration and frequency of gaming lead to the reduction of negative effects that occur due to virtual reality headset usage.

Hypothesis 4: Duration and frequency of gaming with virtual reality headsets lead to the decrease of negative effects due to using.

Hypothesis 5: Employment status of users is a significant factor in diseases that occur due to virtual reality headset usage.

Hypothesis 6: Gender is an important factor in diseases that occur due to virtual reality headset usage.

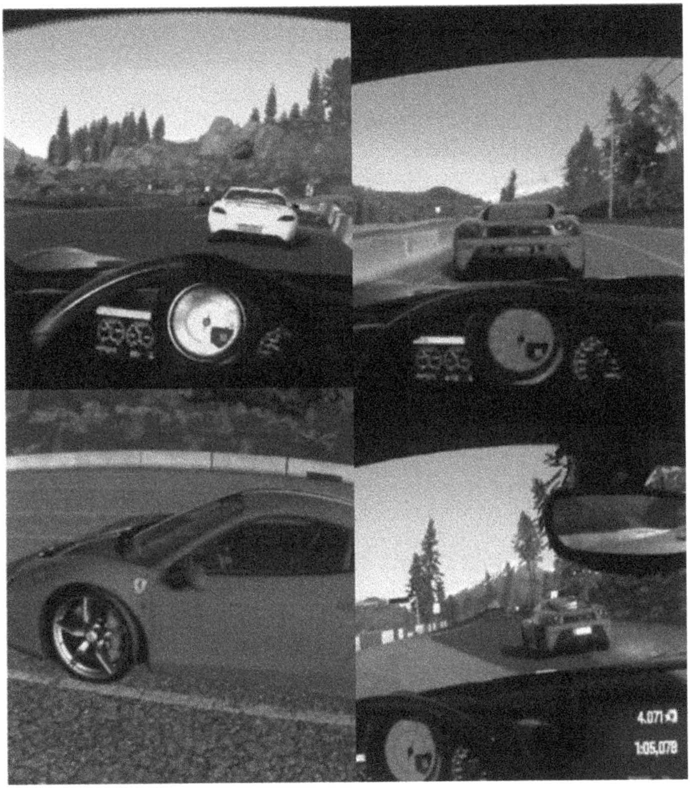

Fig. 8: Images from Drive Club (Driveclub VR, n.d.).

Hypothesis 7: The generally preferred area of users while playing digital games is an important feature in terms of diseases related to using the virtual reality headset.

In the survey questions, outstanding items in studies conducted within the literature were addressed, regarding what are the disturbances felt by users due to virtual reality headset usage. As a result of the reliability test, Cronbach's Alpha value has been observed to be 0.944. The obtained Alpha value shows that the study is reliable enough. Factor analysis was made on existing items, and the following six factors were detected. The obtained KMO and Bartlett's ToS values confirm that the questions are suitable for factor analysis (KMO = 0.653, Bartlett's Test of Sphericity p = 0.000).

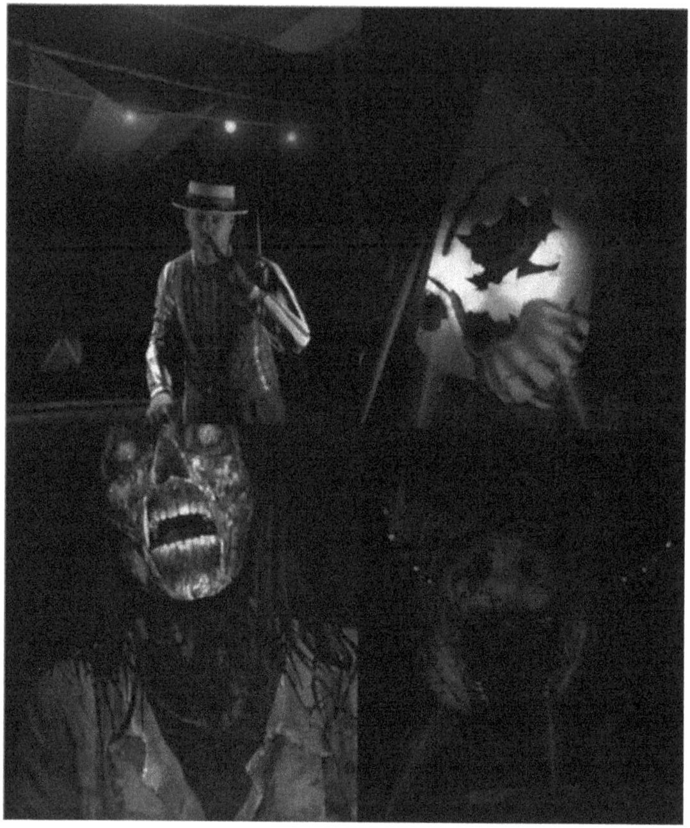

Fig. 9: Images from Until Dawn (Until Down, n.d.).

Six factors are observed in the factor analysis (see Tab. 3). However, when looking at Factor Loads Change Table, it's seen that F1 factor (the percentage of variance = </ex> **41.699**) and F2 factor (the percentage of variance = **12.035** </bx>) are more dominant and distinct in comparison with F3, F4, F5, and F6 factors (see Tab. 4). This situation reveals that "feeling bad due to stomach problems while using a virtual reality headset" and "mental disturbances felt after using a virtual reality headset" are felt more distinctively in comparison with other problems or negative effects.

According to the findings above, **"Virtual reality headsets have negative effects on users"** hypothesis (Hypothesis 1) was accepted.

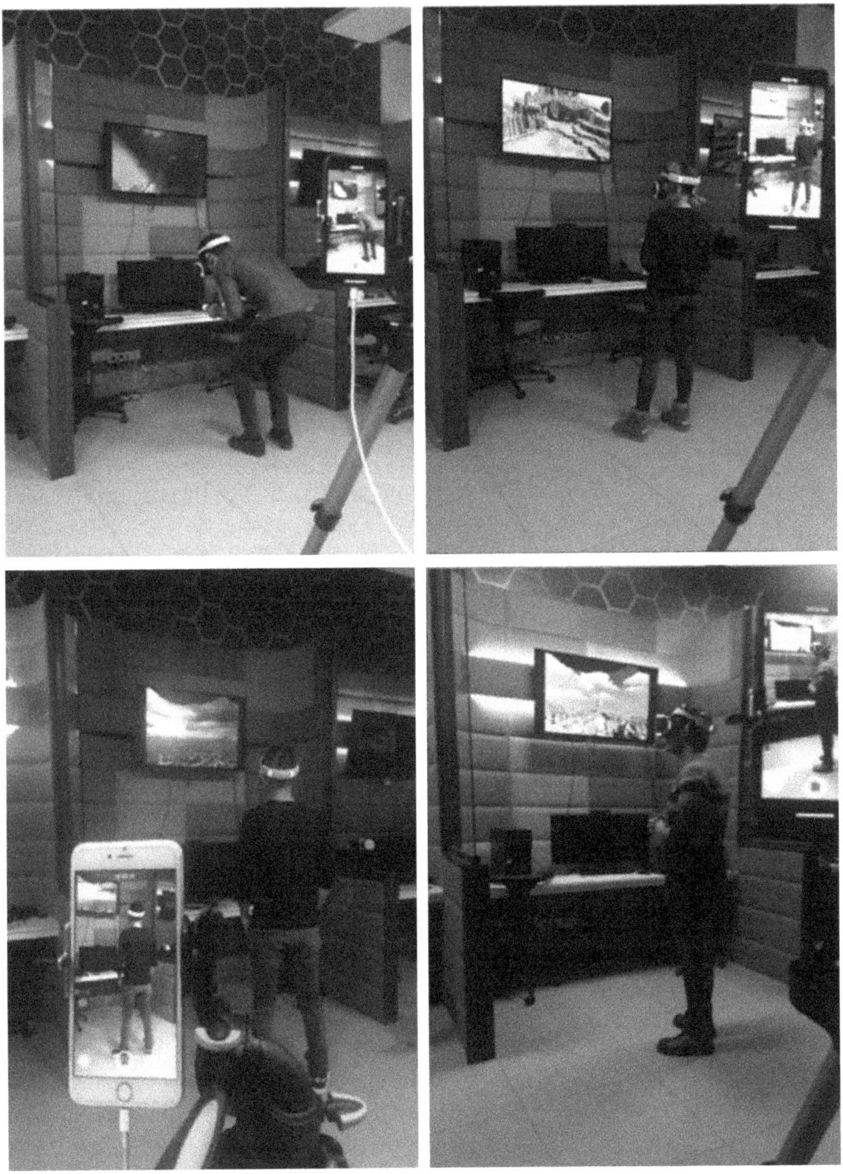

Fig. 10: Visuals from Virtual Reality Study.

Tab. 3: Factors

	1	2	3	4	5	6
F1. "feeling bad due to stomach problems while using a virtual reality headset" factor	**.921**	.069	.210	.072	-.046	.099
	.871	.102	.070	.167	-.014	.097
	.843	.052	.151	.168	.198	.226
	.798	.055	.312	.198	.088	-.052
	.771	.235	.113	.004	.082	.329
	.759	.374	.372	.100	-.052	.092
	.568	.070	.194	.463	.401	.193
F2. "mental disturbance felt after using a virtual reality headset" factor	.168	**.782**	-.019	-.014	.140	.227
	-.018	**.703**	.324	.352	.217	.033
	.079	**.699**	-.039	.150	.218	-.001
	.443	**.639**	.311	.033	-.039	.071
	.352	**.635**	.106	.097	.507	.134
	.110	**.577**	.367	.383	.181	.161
F3. "perspiration felt while using a virtual reality headset" factor	.375	.100	**.784**	.139	.207	.089
	.383	.150	**.764**	.082	.118	.064
	.278	.269	**.614**	.286	.118	.334
F4. "loss of balance felt while using and after using a virtual reality headset" factor	.310	.078	.214	**.745**	.008	.121
	.211	.124	.250	**.730**	.157	.215
	.021	.298	-.115	**.703**	.134	.330
F5. "perception problems felt after using a virtual reality headset" factor	-.078	.219	.206	.373	**.733**	.056
	-.064	.232	.267	-.042	**.723**	.234
	.438	.188	-.143	.106	**.657**	.074
	.005	.459	.211	.113	**.526**	.222
F6. "psychological disturbances felt while using a virtual reality headset" factor	.089	.163	.176	.190	.032	**.797**
	.367	.135	-.083	.277	.246	**.606**
	.259	.011	.466	.166	.257	**.605**
	.182	.159	.071	.436	.264	**.556**

The following have been identified in the descriptive analysis of answers: 52 % of participants are 18–20 years old, 32 % are 21–23 years old, and 16 % are 24 years old and above. All participants (100 %) are single and foundation university students. 14 % of participants are studying journalism, 36 % are studying visual communication design, 82 % are studying public relations and advertising, 10 % are studying radio-television and television journalism programming, and 32 % are studying new media. 42 % of participants spend 0–999 TRY per month, 40 % spend 1000–1999 TRY per month, 16 % spend

Tab. 4: Factor Loads Change

	Total	*Variance Percentage*	*Cumulative Percentage*
F1. "feeling bad due to stomach problems while using a virtual reality headset" factor	11.259	**41.699**	41.699
F2. "mental disturbance felt after using a virtual reality headset" factor	3.249	**12.035**	53.733
F3. "perspiration felt while using a virtual reality headset" factor	1.845	6.835	60.568
F4. "loss of balance felt while using and after using a virtual reality headset" factor	1.492	5.525	66.093
F5. "perception problems felt after using a virtual reality headset" factor	1.252	4.635	70.729
F6. "psychological disturbances felt while using a virtual reality headset" factor	1.032	3.824	74.552

2000–2999 TRY per month, and 2 % spend 3000–3999 TRY per month. 66 % of participants is not employed, 14 % occasionally works on small jobs, 16 % continuously work part-time, and 4 % continuously work full time. 50 % of participants are females, and 50 % are males. While 82 % of participants prefer to be alone while playing digital games, 8 % prefer to be with their families, and 12 % prefer to be in a crowded environment. 12 % of participants have less than 1 year, 10 % have 1–3 years, 14 % have 4–6 years, 26 % have 7–9 years, and 38 % have 10 years or more experience of playing video games. 66 % of participants had their first experience of playing a digital game on a desktop computer, 20 % on a console, 18 % on a mobile device, 12 % on a laptop computer, and 6 % on a tablet. 22 % of participants were 7 years old or younger, 58 % were between 8 and 12 years old, and 20 % were 13 years old or older when they first had a computer. 18 % of participants had their first digital game playing experience between the ages of 5 and 7, 66 % between the ages of 8 and 12, and 16 % when they were 13 or older. 70 % of participants stated that they did not play a game with virtual reality headsets before and 90 % of participants have no virtual reality headsets in their homes.

Inferential analyses were made based on determined factors. These analyses are: Correlation analyses, Mann-Whitney, Kruskal Wallis tests, and median calculations. Analyses were made in terms of educational status, monthly income/expense status, age of first computer obtainment, whether they played games using virtual reality headsets before, class, age, daily duration of playing

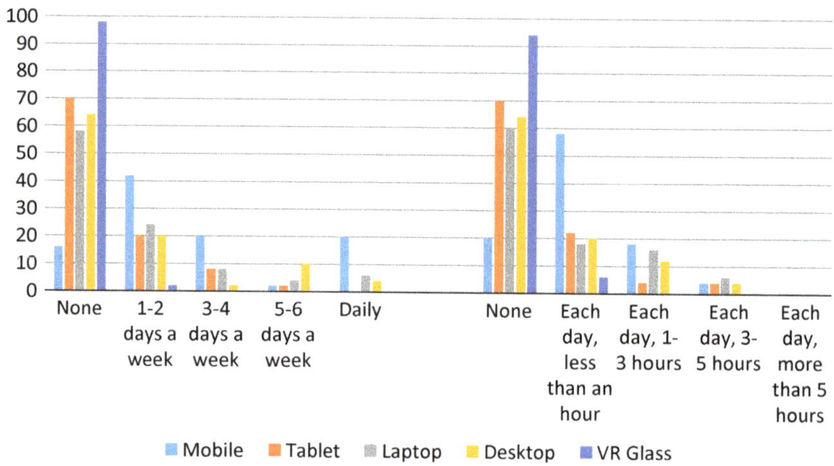

Graphic 1: Digital Gaming Duration (Daily) Frequency (Weekly) Comparison.

digital games on mobile devices and research factors; but no relation was detected. Similarly, analyses were made according to the first genre of digital game played, whether there are virtual reality headsets at home, the type of game that is preferred while playing with virtual reality headsets at home; but no significant difference was detected.

The participants have been asked how often they play digital games on a weekly basis with a mobile device, tablet, laptop, desktop and virtual reality headsets; and how long they play digital games on a daily basis. Their responses have been visualized in the Graphic 1.

Accordingly, it is seen that participants play digital games 1–2 days a week and 1–2 hours a day on mobile devices, tablets, laptops, and desktop computers. It is seen that weekly and daily gaming rates are pretty low when it comes to virtual reality headsets.

58 % of participants play digital games on a mobile device every day even for less than 1 hour; the rate is 22 % for the ones answering the same question for tablets, 20 % for desktops, 18 % for laptops, and only 6 % for virtual reality headsets.

16 % of the participants stated that they never play digital games on mobile devices weekly; the rate is 58 % for the ones answering the same question for laptops, 64 % for desktops, 70 % for tablets, and 98 % for virtual reality headsets.

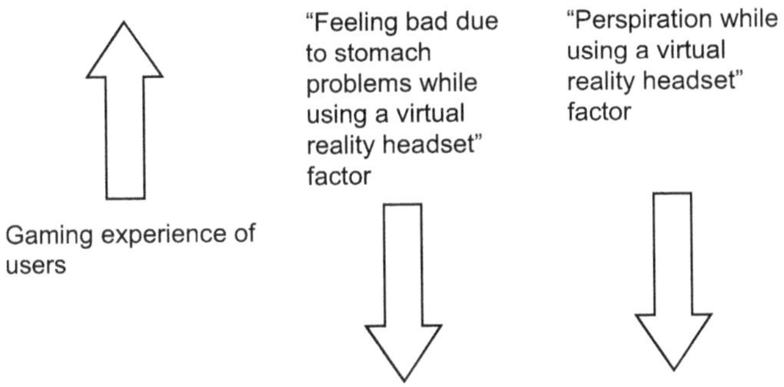

Fig. 11: The Relationship Between Gaming Experience of Users and Virtual Reality Headset Related Symptoms.

According to those findings, **"Virtual reality headsets don't have widespread use within the scope of digital gaming experience yet"** hypothesis (Hypothesis 2) was accepted.

There is a negative relationship between gaming experience of users and "feeling bad due to stomach problems while using virtual reality headsets" factor (rho =-0.352, p = 0.012). There is a negative relationship between gaming experience of users and "perspiration while using virtual reality headsets" factor (rho =-0.348, p = 0.013) (see Fig. 11). The generated situation shows that stomach problems and perspiration due to using virtual reality headsets decrease as duration and frequency of gaming experience increase.

There is a negative relationship between the daily digital gaming duration of participants on a laptop and the "feeling bad due to stomach problems while using a virtual reality headset" factor (rho = -0.280 p = 0.049). There is a negative relationship between the daily digital gaming duration of participants on a laptop and the "psychological disturbances felt while using a virtual reality headset" factor (rho = -0.281 p = 0.048) (see Fig. 12).

There is a negative relationship between daily digital gaming duration of participants on desktop computers and "perspiration while using a virtual reality headset" factor (rho= -0.421 p=0.002). There is a negative relationship between daily digital gaming duration of participants on desktop computers and "psychological disturbances felt while using a virtual reality headset" factor (rho= -0.306 p=0.031) (see Fig. 13).

There is a negative relationship between weekly digital gaming frequency of participants on desktop computers and "perspiration while using a virtual reality headset" factor (rho= -0.440 p=0.001). There is a negative relationship

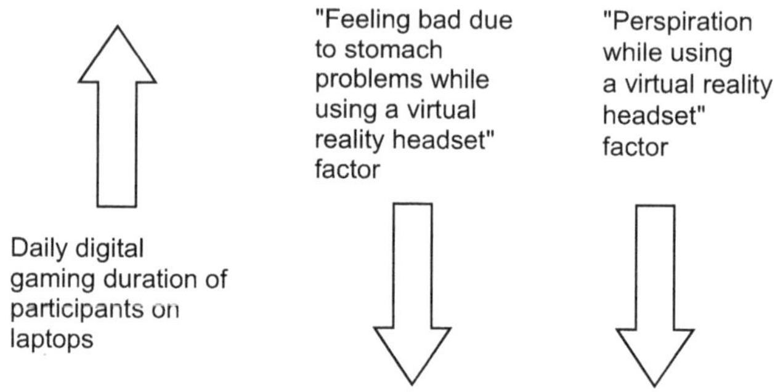

Fig. 12: The Relationship Between Daily Digital Gaming Duration of Participants on Laptops and Symptoms Related to Using Virtual Reality Headsets.

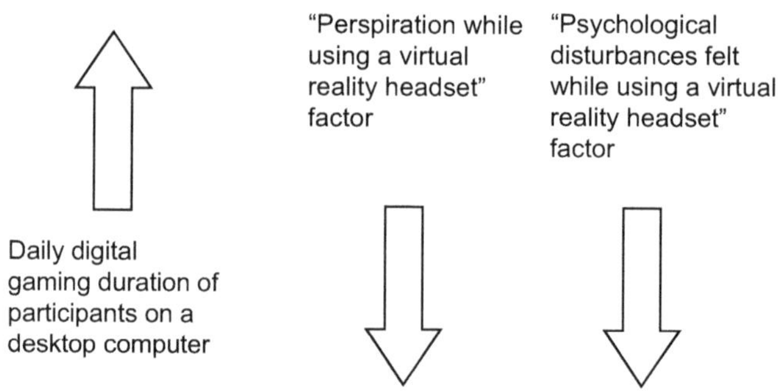

Fig. 13: The Relationship Between Daily Digital Gaming Duration of Participants on Desktop Computers and Symptoms Related to Using Virtual Reality Headsets.

between weekly digital gaming frequency of participants on desktop computers and "loss of balance felt during and after using a virtual reality headset" factor (rho= -0.287 p=0.043). There is a negative relationship between weekly digital gaming frequency of participants on desktop computers and "psychological disturbances felt while using a virtual reality headset" factor (rho= -0.295 p=0.038) (see Fig. 14).

According to these findings, **"Gamer experience formed by the duration and frequency of digital gaming on other media lead to the reduction of negative effects that occur due to using virtual reality headsets"** hypothesis (Hypothesis 3) was accepted. However, if that player experience has developed as a result of the games played by virtual reality headsets, one of the negative effects

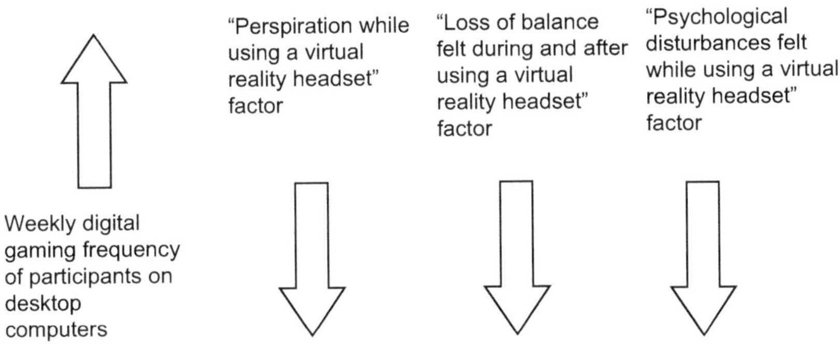

Fig. 14: The Relationship Between Weekly Digital Gaming Frequency of Participants on Desktop Computers and Symptoms Related to Using Virtual Reality Headsets.

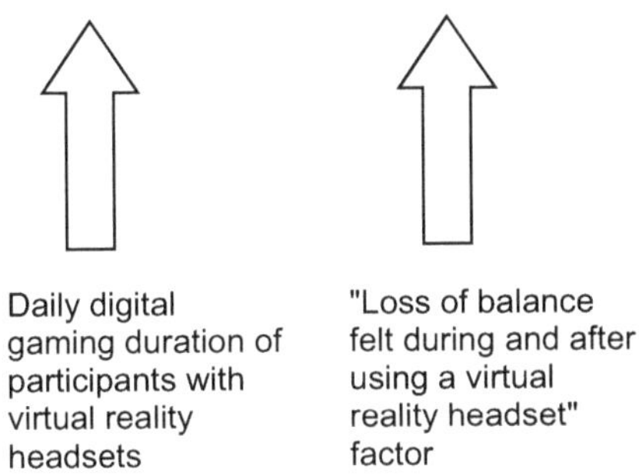

Fig. 15: The Relationship Between Daily Digital Gaming Duration of Participants with Virtual Reality Headsets and Symptoms Related to Using Virtual Reality Headsets.

triggered by the use of virtual reality, loss of balance, has not decreased, but increased. There is a positive relationship between daily digital gaming duration of participants with virtual reality headsets and weekly digital gaming frequency of participants with virtual reality headsets (rho=0.565 p=0.000). There is a positive relationship between daily digital gaming duration of participants and "loss of balance felt during and after using a virtual reality headset" factor (rho=0.322 p=0.022) (see Fig. 15).

There is a negative relationship between employment statuses of participants and "feeling bad due to stomach problems while using a virtual reality headset" factor (rho= -0.488 p=0.000). There is a negative relationship between employment statuses of participants and "mental disturbances felt after using a virtual

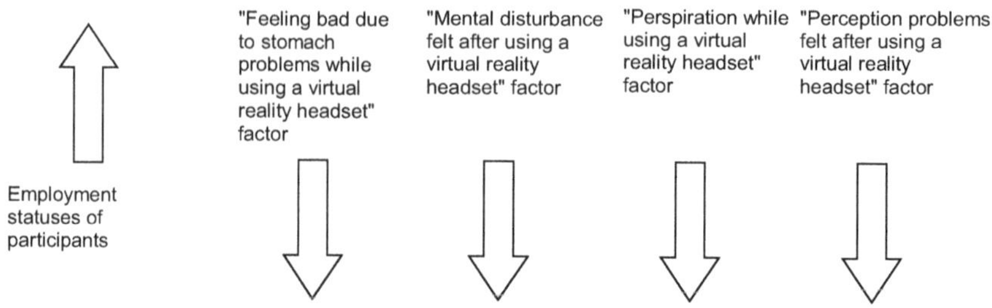

Fig. 16: The Relationship Between Employment Statuses of Participants and Diseases Related to Using Virtual Reality Headsets.

reality headset" factor (rho= -0.444 p=0.001). There is a negative relationship between employment statuses of participants and "perspiration while using a virtual reality headset" factor (rho= -0.488 p=0.001). There is a negative relationship between employment statuses of participants and "perception disturbances felt after using a virtual reality headset" factor (rho= -0.321 p=0.023) (see Fig. 16).

As employment statuses of participants increase, in other words, as their participation to real life increases, they seem to be affected less by stomach problems, mental disturbances, perspiration, and perception disturbances felt due to using virtual reality headsets. According to those findings, **"Employment status of users is a significant factor in diseases that occur due to virtual reality headset usage"** hypothesis (Hypothesis 5) was accepted.

There was a significant difference between genders of participants in terms of " feeling bad due to stomach problems while using a virtual reality headset" factor (Mean rank Women=31.90, Men=19.10, p=0.001). It is seen that women feel stomach problems that occur due to using a virtual reality headset more than men. There was a significant difference between genders of participants in terms of "perspiration while using a virtual reality headset" factor (Mean rank Women=34.18, Men=16.82, p=0.000). It is seen that women feel more perspiration/heat than men while using a virtual reality headset. There was a significant difference between genders of participants in terms of "loss of balance felt during and after using a virtual reality headset" factor (Mean rank Women=31.76, Men=19.24, p=0.002). It is seen that women feel more loss of balance than men while using a virtual reality headset. There was a significant difference between genders of participants in terms of "psychological differences felt while using a virtual reality headset" factor (Mean rank Women=30.36, Men=20.64, p=0.017). It is seen that women feel more psychological disturbances than men while using a virtual reality headset. Accordingly, it is seen that gender is an important

Tab. 5: According to Research Factors Preference of Environment While Playing Digital Games

	F1	F2	F3	F4	F5	F6
Alone						
Valid	41	41	41	41	41	41
Missing Value	0	0	0	0	0	0
Median	1.00	1.50	2.00	**3.00**	1.50	2.50
With Family						
Valid	4	4	4	4	4	4
Missing Value	0	0	0	0	0	0
Median	2.50	2.00	4.00	3.00	2.00	**4.50**
In a Crowded Environment						
Valid	6	6	6	6	6	6
Missing Value	0	0	0	0	0	0
Median	1.00	1.00	300	3.50	1.50	**4.00**

demographic characteristic in terms of negative effects that occur due to using a virtual reality headset.

According to these findings, **"Gender is an important factor in diseases that occur due to virtual reality headset usage"** hypothesis (Hypothesis 6) was accepted.

Within the scope of the research, median values of digital gaming environment preference information were calculated according to factor means. Accordingly, it is seen that those who prefer to be alone while playing digital games are susceptible to "loss of balance felt during and after using a virtual reality headset" factor the most, while those who prefer to be with family or in a crowded environment while playing digital games are susceptible to "psychological disturbances felt while using a virtual reality headset" factor the most (see Tab. 5).

According to these findings, **"The preferred area of users while playing digital games, is an important feature in terms of diseases related using the virtual reality headset"** hypothesis (Hypothesis 7) was accepted.

The Frequency Distribution of the Symptoms Related to Virtual Reality Headset Use

In the questionnaire study, the participants have been asked several symptoms and to mark the choices based on the five-point Likert scale in terms of how much they feel them. According to their responses, the most felt symptoms or psychological situations have been listed in Tab. 6. In the table, it is stated which sets Kennedy (1993) developed for Simulator Sickness Questionnaire (Oculomotor, Disorientation, Nausea) the symptoms are included in. No coding has been made for the symptoms or psychological situations that cannot be counted in any sets.

Considering only the ones that can be set to cluster coding from the symptoms listed in this table, the prevalence of the symptom sets was as follows: (1) Orientation disorder, (2) nausea (3) oculomotor. The results were consistent with Stanney et al. (1997: 1138)'s symptom dominance set for virtual environment disease.

The rates of the participants who had to terminate the use of virtual reality headsets because they felt very severe symptoms were also determined. The Eagle Flight game, which is an action game and played in the "FPS, First Person Shooter" way, was played for 5 minutes to each participant, and no participants ended the virtual reality experience due to severe symptoms in those 5 minutes. In the Robots Rescue game, which is an action game and played in the "Role Playing" way, 2 % of the participants; in the Drive Club game, which is an action game and played in the FPS way, 4 % of the participants; and in the Until Dawn game which is a horror game played in the FPS way, 6 % of the participants ended virtual reality experience due to severe symptoms.

Conclusion

With the advance of technology, communication tools are also being updated and constantly renewed. The effects of these renewed or recently introduced communication tools on users are thus studied. These effects define the future of new communication technologies. It is likely that technology of virtual reality will transform into a more common communication platform as that technology becomes more economical. In this study, symptoms induced by virtual reality and the factors that affect those symptoms have been studied. This subject is closely related to the future of virtual reality applications.

It has been observed that in the technological development, VR users, together with simulators, also experience the motion sickness symptoms related to physical reality. Initially, those sicknesses in that new technology were regarded as motion sickness seen in simulator environment and triggered by VR. However, because of the differences in both symptoms and trigger mechanisms, new nomenclatures have been made as simulator sickness and cybersickness.

Although there have been several theories about and numerous studies on how that sickness has occurred so far, the problem still exists. On the one hand, these

Tab. 6: The Prevalence of the Symptoms

Symptoms	Strongly disagree	Disagree	Uncertain	Agree	Strongly agree	Agree and strongly agree
Loss of balance (Disorientation)	18	10	18	30	24	**54**
Tension	14	12	22	28	24	**52**
Sweating (Nausea)	24	14	12	26	24	**50**
Over excitement	10	18	23	35	14	**49**
Heat, sweating	22	20	14	28	16	**44**
Drowsiness	24	28	16	22	20	**42**
Dizzy (Disorientation)	20	23	18	21	18	**39**
Uneasiness	28	20	26	14	12	**26**
Cold sweating	44	20	14	10	12	**22**
Anxiety	36	28	15	8	13	**21**
Headache (Oculomotor)	52	20	8	10	10	**20**
General discomfort (Nausea and Oculomotor)	50	23	8	13	6	**19**
Fatigue (Oculomotor)	34	20	28	12	6	**18**
Nausea (Nausea and Disorientation)	54	22	8	6	10	**16**
Stomach awareness (Nausea)	64	16	4	10	6	**16**
Lethargy	48	26	10	10	6	**16**
Photophobia, sensitivity to light (Oculomotor)	41	31	12	16	0	**16**
Difficulty concentration (Nausea and Oculomotor)	43	31	12	6	8	**14**
Sensitive stomach	52	24	12	4	8	**12**
Feeling that "everything is moving"	60	26	4	4	6	**10**
Flashes of light in head	66	20	4	8	2	**10**
Eye burning, ache, watering (Oculomotor)	54	28	12	2	4	**6**

theories provide valid arguments. On the other hand, it is also observed that there are some questions those theories have failed to respond to. No consensus can be reached on how the sickness has occurred. Additionally, personal differences for susceptibility to motion sickness have not been understood exactly. Besides, these theories are not strong enough to anticipate or estimate the sickness.

VR applications penetrate all areas of technological world ranging from education to medicine, from industry to scientific researches and from entertainment to video games market. Cybersickness is one of the most significant health and safety issues that might affect the progress of virtual environment technology. Even though the theories put forward and studies done have not been able to eliminate the problem completely, a sort of guide has been provided and will continue to provide for designers and coders of cyberspace systems to show them which methods and how to use those methods. In other words, studies cannot eliminate the problem, but they make a serious contribution to the comprehensive understanding of the problem.

In this study, 50 participants who played four (4) different VR games in Istanbul Aydın University Laboratory have been asked 52 questions selected from Motion Sickness Questionnaire and Simulator Sickness Questionnaire, as well as symptoms specifically identified for this study and demographic questions. The symptoms correlated with the clusters created for Kennedy's (1993) Simulator Sickness Questionnaire have been coded as "oculomotor, disorientation, nausea". The symptoms reported by the participants are as follows according to the prevalence: loss of balance *(disorientation)*, tension, sweating *(nausea)*, over excitement, heat, sweating, drowsiness, dizzy *(disorientation)*, uneasiness, cold sweating, anxiety, headache *(oculomotor)*, general discomfort *(nausea and oculomotor)*, fatigue *(oculomotor)*, nausea *(nausea and oculomotor)*, stomach awareness *(nausea)*, lethargy, photophobia *(oculomotor)*, difficulty concentration *(nausea and oculomotor)*, sensitive stomach, feeling that "everything is moving", flashes of light in head, eye burning, ache, and watering *(oculomotor)*.

When only the symptoms that can be coded as clusters are considered, the prevalence of symptom sets are the following: (1) disorientation, (2) nausea (3) oculomotor. The symptoms have demonstrated a correlation with Stanney et al. (1997: 1138)'s prevalence of symptom dominance clusters.

When a factor analysis has been conducted for all symptoms asked in the questionnaire, six factors have been determined. If the percentage changes of factor loading are examined, it can be seen that the first two factors are more dominant. The symptom groups have been listed accordingly based on dominance degree: "stomach problem while using a virtual reality headset", "mental disorder after using a virtual reality headset", "sweating while using a virtual reality headset", "loss of balance during and after using a virtual reality headset", "perception problem after using a virtual reality headset", and "psychological disorders while using a virtual reality headset". Although the player experience provided by virtual reality headsets is interesting, it can be seen that negative effects because of use of them are also experienced.

The rates of users who had to end the use of virtual reality headsets because of very severe symptoms have also been identified. The action game Eagle Flight, which is played as "FPS, First Person Shooter", was played for 5 minutes, and no one ended the virtual reality experience because of severe symptoms during those 5 minutes. As for the action game Robots Rescue, which is played as "Role Playing", 2 % of participants ended the virtual reality experience because of severe symptoms. This rate is 4 % for the action game Drive Club, which is played as FPS and 6 % for the horror game Until Dawn, which is played as FPS. As can be seen, the rate of participants who could not complete the virtual reality experience because of severe symptoms is the highest for the horror type game.

Inferential analysis has also been conducted in the study. The educational status, monthly income/expenses, first age of getting a computer of the participant, whether he or she has ever played a game using a virtual reality headset or not, class, age, and the duration of playing digital games with a mobile device daily have been considered within the study factors and made parts of analysis. However, no correlation has been identified. Similarly, analysis has also been conducted in accordance with the department at the university—the first game type played, whether there is a virtual reality headset at home or not, the preferred game type played with a virtual reality headset at home—but no significant difference has been identified.

As the player's experience due to the duration and frequency of other digital game playing increases, the negative effects resulting from the use of virtual reality headsets decreases. However, if that player's experience has developed as a result of the games played by virtual reality headsets, one of the negative effects triggered by the use of virtual reality, loss of balance, has not decreased, but increased. There is a positive correlation between the participants' duration of digital game playing with virtual reality headsets and "loss of balance felt during and after the use of virtual reality headset".

As the employment status of the participants increases, that is to say, their professional experiences in real life increase, it has been observed that they have been affected less by stomach disorder, mental disorder, sweating, and perception disorder felt because of the use of virtual reality headsets. Sex is also an important demographic feature on the negative effects felt as a result of the use of virtual reality headsets. Women have experienced more serious stomach disorders, sweating, feeling hot, and loss of balance because of the use of virtual reality headsets than men have. The setting that the participants prefer when they play digital games is also effective on the negative effects resulted from the use of virtual reality headsets. It has been observed that the ones who prefer to be alone when they play digital games are more susceptible to "loss of balance felt during and after the use of virtual reality headsets", while the ones who prefer to be with their families or in a crowded place are more susceptible to "psychological disorders felt during the use of virtual reality headsets".

It is likely that virtual reality technology used for short periods now by users will become a daily life practice like driving a car or watching TV. However, the biggest obstacle for that to happen is the negative effects and symptoms triggered by virtual reality. For the frequency and severity of those symptoms to decrease, more research on this matter is needed. However, no consensus has been reached so far on any theory that can explain why cybersickness occurs and that can anticipate its symptoms.

Bibliography

Barrett, J. (2004). Side Effects of Virtual Environments: A Review of the Literature. Edinburgh Australia: DSTO Information Sciences Laboratory.

Bouchard, S., Robillard, G. and Renaud, P. (2007). Revising the Factor Structure of the Simulator Sickness Questionnaire. Annual Review of Cybertherapy and Telemedicine, 5(Summer), 128–137.

Braithwaite, M. G. and Braithwaite, B. D. (1990). Simulator Sickness in an Army Simulator. Journal of the Society of Occupational Medicine, 40, 105–110.

Brooks, J. O., Goodenough, R. R., Crisler, M. C., Klein, N. D., Alley, R. L., Koon, B. L. and Wills, R. F. (2010). Simulator Sickness During Driving Simulation Studies. Accident Analysis & Prevention, 42(3), 788–796.

Büyükkurt, S., Demir, S. C., Özgünen, F. T., Evrüke, İ. C., Kadayıfçı, O. and Güzel, A. B. (2008). Gebelikte Bulantı-Kusma Yakınması Olan Hastanın Değerlendirilmesi ve Tedavi Seçenekleri. Türkiye Klinikleri Journal of Gynecology and Obstetrics, 18(2), 106–116.

Calvert, S. and Tan, S. (1994). Impact of Virtual Reality on Young Adults' Physiological Arousal and Aggressive Thoughts: Interaction versus Observation. Journal of Applied Developmental Psychology, 15(1), 125–139.

Claremont, C. A. (1931). The Psychology of Seasickness. Psyche, 11, 86–90.

Cobb, S., Nichols, S., Ramsey, A. and Wilson, J. R. (1999). Virtual Reality-Induced Symptoms and Effects (VRISE). Presence: Teleoperators and Virtual Environments, 8(2), 169–186.

Costello, P. J. (1997). Health and Safety Issues Associated with Virtual Reality: A Review of Current Literature (pp. 1–23). Loughborough, UK: Advisory Group on Computer Graphics.

Dağtaş, B. (1994). Kullanma ve Etki Modeli. In B. Dağtaş & U. Demiray (Eds.), Kitle İletişim Çalışmaları İçin İletişim Modelleri (pp.125–129). Eskişehir: T.C. Anadolu Üniversitesi Yayınları.

DriveclubVR. (n.d.) Retrieved from https://www.playstation.com/tr-tr/games/driveclub-vr-ps4/ on 18 September 2018.

Duh, H. B.-L., Lin, J. J.W., Kenyon, R. V., Parker, D. E. and Furness, T. A. (2002). Effects of Characteristics of Image Quality in an Immersive Environment. Presence: Teleoperators and Virtual Environments, 11(3), 324–332.

Duh, H. B.-L., Parker, D. E., Philips, J. O. and Furness, T. A. (2004). "Conflicting" Motion Cues to the Visual and Vestibular Self-motion Systems around 0.06 Hz Evoke Simulator Sickness. Human Factors, 46(1), 142–153.

Eagle Flight. (n.d.). Retrieved from https://store.playstation.com/tr-tr/product/EP0001-CUSA04876_00-EAGLEFLIGHTGAME0 on 12 September 2018.

Gianaros, P. J., Muth, E. R., Mordkoff, J. T., Levine, M. E. and Stern, R. M. (2001). A Questionnaire for the Assessment of the Multiple Dimensions of Motion Sickness. Aviation, Space, and Environmental Medicine, 72(2), 115–119.

Golding, J. F. (2006). Motion Sickness Susceptibility. Autonomic Neuroscience: Basic and Clinical, 129, 67–76.

Graybiel, A. (1988). Motion Sickness. In J.M. Wolfe (Ed.), Sensory Systems: II (pp. 44–46). Boston: Birkhäuser.

Highstein, S. M. (2004). Anatomy and Physiology of the Central and Peripheral Vestibular System: Overview. In S.M. Highstein, R.R. Fay & A.N. Popper (Eds.), The Vestibular System (pp. 1–10). New York: Springer.

Howarth, P. A. and Finch, M. (1999). The Nauseogenicity of Two Methods of Navigating Within a Virtual Environment. Applied Ergonomics, 30(1), 39–45.

Irwin, J. A. (1881). Preliminary Observations on the Pathology of Sea-sickness. Ballantyne: Hanson & Company.

Johnson, D. M. (2005). Introduction to and Review of Simulator Sickness Research. Research Report 1832, U.S. Army Research Institute for the Behavioural and Social Sciences. Arlington, Virginia.

Kemeny, A. (2014). From Driving Simulation to Virtual Reality. Proceedings of the Laval Virtual Reality International Conference (pp. 1–5). Laval, France.

Kennedy, R. S., Berbaum, K. S., Lilienthal, M. G., Dunlap, W. P., Mulligan, B. F. and Funaro, J. F. (1987). Guidelines for Alleviation of Simulator Sickness Symptomatology. Orlando, Florida: Naval Training Systems Center.

Kennedy, R.S., Lane, N.E. Berbaun, K.S. Lilienthal, M.G. (1993). Simulator Sickness Questionnaire: An Enhanced Method for Quantifying Simulator Sickness. The International Journal of Aviation Psychology, 3(3), 203–220.

Kolasinski, E. M. (1995). Simulator Sickness in Virtual Environments. Technical Report (No. ARI-TR-1027), Virginia: U.S. Army Research Institute for the Behavioral and Social Sciences.

Koslucher, F., Haaland, E., Malsch, A., Webeler, J. and Stoffregen, T. A. (2015). Sex Differences in the Incidence of Motion Sickness Induced by Linear Visual Oscillation. Aerospace Medicine and Human Performance, 86(9), 787–793.

Lampton, D. R., Kolasinski, E. M., Knerr, B. W., Bliss, J. P., Bailey, J. H. and Witmer, B. G. (1994). Side Effects and Aftereffects of Immersion in Virtual Environments. Proceedings of the Human Factors and Ergonomics Society 38th Annual Meeting (pp. 1154–1157).

LaViola, J. J. (2000). A Discussion of Cybersickness in Virtual Environments. Technical Report, Brown University Providence, SIGCHI Bulletin, 32(1), 47–56.

Lawson, B. D. (2014). Motion Sickness Symptomatology and Origins. In S.H. Kelly & K.M. Stanney (Eds.), Handbook of Virtual Environment: Design, Implementation, and Applications (pp. 531–600). Boca Raton: CRC Press.

Lawson, B. D., Graeber, D. A., Mead, A. M. and Muth, E. R. (2002). Signs and Symptoms of Human Syndromes Associated with Synthetic Experiences. In K.M. Stanney (Ed.), Handbook of Virtual Environment: Design, Implementation and Applications (pp. 589–618). New Jersey: Lawrence Erlbaum Associates Publishers.

Lin, J. W., Duh, H. B.-L., Parker, D. E., Abi-Rached, H. and Furness, T. A. (2002). Effects of Field of View on Presence, Enjoyment, Memory, and Simulator Sickness in a Virtual Environment. Proceedings of the IEEE Virtual Reality Annual International Symposium (pp. 164–171). Orlando, Florida.

Lu, D. (2016). Virtual Reality sickness during immersion: An investigation of potential obstacles towards general accessibility of VR technology (Master Thesis, Uppsala University, Uppsala, Sweden) Retrieved from https://www.diva-portal.org/smash/get/diva2:1129675/FULLTEXT01.pdf on 13 December 2017

McCauley, M. E. and Sharkey, T. J. (1992). Cybersickness: Perception of Self-Motion in Virtual Environments. Presence: Teleoperators & Virtual Environments, 1(3), 311–318.

Munafo, J., Diedrick, M. and Stoffregen, T. A. (2017). The Virtual Reality Head-Mounted Display Oculus Rift Induces Motion Sickness and is Sexist in Its Effects. Experimental Brain Research, 235(3), 889–901.

Nichols, S., Ramsey, A. D., Cobb, S., Neale, H., D'Cruz, M. and Wilson, J. R. (2000). Incidence of Virtual Reality Symptoms and Effects (VRISE) in Desktop and Projection Screen Displays. Sudbury Norwich: HSE Books.

Oman, C. M. (1991). Sensory Conflict in Motion Sickness: An Observer Theory Approach. In S. Ellis (Ed.), Pictorial Communication in Real and Virtual Environments (pp. 362–376). London: Taylor and Francis.

Oman, C. M. (1998). Sensory Conflict Theory and Space Sickness: Our Changing Perspective. Journal of Vestibular Research, 8(1), 5 I–56.

Park, G. D., Allen, R.W., Fiorentino, D., Rosenthal, T. J. and Cook, M. L. (2006). Simulator Sickness Scores According to Symptom Susceptibility, Age, and Gender for an Older Driver Assessment Study. Proceedings of the Human Factors and Ergonomics Society Annual Meeting, 50(26), 2702–2706.

Reason, J. T. (1978). Motion Sickness Adaptation: A Neural Mismatch Model. Journal of the Royal Society of Medicine, 71(11), 819.

Regan, E. C. and Price, K. R. (1993a). Some Side Effects of Immersion Virtual Reality in a Population of Firefighters. APRE working paper, 9/93.

Regan, E. C. and Price, K. R. (1993b). Subjective Views on an Immersion Virtual Reality System and Its Peripherals. APRE Working paper, 16/93.

Riccio, G. E. and Stoffregen, T. A. (1991). An Ecological Theory of Motion Sickness and Postural Instability. Ecological Psychology, 3(3), 195–240.

Sharples, S. Cobb, S., Moody, A. and Wilson, J. R. (2008). Virtual Reality Induced Symptoms and Effects (VRISE): Comparison of Head Mounted Display (HMD), Desktop and Projection Display Systems. Displays, 29(2), 58–69.

Smith, D. (2019, May 21). PlayStation VR is my favorite new party trick. Insider [Image]. Retrieved from https://www.insider.com/playstation-vr-review-ps4-2019-3 on 30 May 2019.

Stanney, K. M. (2002). Handbook of Virtual Environments. London: Lawrence Erlbaum Associates Publishers.

Stanney, K. M., Kennedy, R. S. and Drexler, J. M. (1997). Cybersickness is not Simulator Sickness. Proceedings of the Human Factors and Ergonomics Society 41st Annual Meeting (pp. 1138–1142). Albuquerque, New Mexico, USA.

Stanney, K. M., Mourant, R. R. and Kennedy, R. S. (1998). Human Factors Issues in Virtual Environments: A Review of the Literature. Presence: Teleoperators and Virtual Environments Archive, 7(4), 327–351.

Stoffregen, T. A., Chang, C-H., Chen, F-C. and Zeng, W-J. (2017). Effects of Decades of Physical Driving on Body Movement and Motion Sickness During Virtual Driving. PLoS ONE, 12(11). e0187120. DOI: https://doi.org/10.1371/journal.pone.0187120

Strickland, D. and Cartier, D. (1997). EEG Measurements in a Virtually Reality Headset, Presence: Teleoperators and Virtual Environments, 6(5), 581–589.

Tekinalp, Ş. and Uzun, R. (2009). İletişim Araştırmaları ve Kuramları. İstanbul: Beta Basım.

The Nirvanist (2016, Jul 22). Off the Bench and into the Game: PSVR. Virtual reality Pop [Image]. Retrieved from https://virtualrealitypop.com/off-the-bench-and-into-the-game-psvr-bf8aa07145fb on 12 April 2017.

The VR Playroom. (n.d.). Retrieved from https://store.playstation.com/tr-tr/product/IP9100-CUSA04318_00-EU00000000000000 on 10 October 2018.

Torre, J. (2014, March 19). #Sony presenta sus lentes de realidad virtual para #PS4 El Project Morpheus [Image]. Retrieved from http://johnnytorre.blogspot.com/2014_03_16_archive.html on 12 April 2017.

Treisman. M. (1977). Motion Sickness: An Evolutionary Hypothesis. Science, 197, 493–495.

Until Down: Rush of Blood. (n.d.). Retrieved from https://store.playstation.com/tr-tr/product/EP9000-CUSA02350_00-RUSHOFBLOOD00001 on 23 September 2018

Uzun, R. (2013). İzleyici Merkezli Yaklaşımlar. In E. Yüksel (Ed.), İletişim Kuramları (pp. 84–105). Eskişehir: T.C. Anadolu Üniversitesi Yayınları.

Ayten Övür

Digital Ecstasy as Escapist Fantasy Field in the Age of Technology

Abstract: This study illuminates the digital ecstasy experienced by the human communities that have lost their interest and perception for the outside world, that have isolated themselves from the real life like sleepwalkers, and, as a result, have dived into virtual lives and fantasies. Digital ecstasy refers to the condition of being ecstatic and numbed under the effects of simulations and fantasies emerged by developed technologies. Even though the reasons of digital ecstasy might show similarities with the effects of alcohol, drunkenness caused by alcohol gives one a sort of relieving feeling that might make one forget some desires. However, in digital ecstasy, instead of forgetting those desires, materializing them even virtually and achieving satisfaction is important. This study, from the perspective of uses and gratifications approach, examines our relationship with social media that was initially used as a leisure time activity and to erase our boredom, but has gradually turned into a sort of duty that requires us to study hard and to overexert for it.

Keywords: digital ecstasy, virtual lives, escapist fantasy, catharsis

Introduction

People's attitudes, behaviors and habits have been changing in our era where we have become more and more addicted to the social media, digital games and any information on the internet; and most of the people include those white-collar who work in front of a computer. We are surrounded by people who have lost interest in the outer world and dived into virtual worlds and fantasias, looking just like sleepwalkers.

As the number of people who does not live for the moment but instead try to make an unreal copy out of it is increasing, one famous saying "Carpe Diem[1]" becomes more meaningful. Those who are in digital ecstasy[2] in which they are disconnected emotionally from the moment and place they are actually in see events and facts around themselves as potential materials to be used in their

1 Carpe diem is a Latin aphorism, usually translated "seize the day", taken from book 1 of the Roman poet Horace's work Odes (23 BC). Meaning enjoy the moment. (Wikipedia)

2 Inebriation: The state or characteristic of drunkenness. To open the gates of consciousness through a drug substance. As a result, losing physical and mental control is dangerous as it creates addiction. (Ekşisözlük)

virtual world, and this means taking away from the importance, value and meaning of reality. Throughout the history, people have kept their imaginations and minds with various fantasias, taken shelter in or idle around fanciful events. In today's virtual reality and technology world, however, our fantasias have reached another dimension. Fantasias with vivid images and visuals, almost same as the real ones, have been trying to cross the line of virtual world and overflow into the real world. Our fantasias have been one step closer to the reality with technologies such as artificial intelligence, hologram and virtual reality glasses.

Once only imagined with books, our fantasias started to talk via radio and was pictured via television and has become three dimensional via virtual reality. As our fantasias are getting one step closer to reality with each new technology, people are getting more influenced and lost within this ecstasy. Why we are more involved with digital ecstasy each and every day is something that today's researchers should focus on. In this chapter, reasons and outcomes of digital ecstasy regarding psychology will be studied.

Virtual Reality

Technology has been transforming the social life. Harold Adam Innis and Marshal McLuhan who study this transformation say that technology change the way people think, make choice and even live. The human being who is an individual of techno-social life, making a techno-copy out of real life and turning it into a part of their life, has moved onto a new phase where virtual reality and real life are interlaced. Innis and McLuhan have seen technology, which is referred as a solution of world's problems, as a structure which is definitely partial and serving the dominant powers (as cited in Yengin ve Bayrak, 2017: 41–44).

Even though technology was a controlling effort aiming to develop certain production techniques and products in the beginning, this has changed. Technology has been both changing and being changed. The pain of change has affected those who made and has been making this change. Although it is late, thinkers and culture commentators all around the world have been trying to explicate technology. It does not seem possible to make a sense of our lives without understanding technology first. We are in the effort to sense the change and to supervise those supervisors who we assume to be supervising on us (İnam, 2014: 21).

Internet is sheltering and risk-free yet also a center of attraction for the youth with its structure characterized as reformist and nonhierarchical. People can realize their search for novelty and desire for freedom on the internet with their virtual identities via which they can express themselves virtually without having to bear responsibility. So-called alternative social spaces to real life has been created with categories such as discussions, entertainment and searching for friends on the internet; and young people have been offered with illusory active role with a single type of entertainment fostered by the consumption culture (Söğüt, 2015: 165). It is seen that, today, network of technology-based relationships has started to settle and that they are maintained without meeting, sometimes via social media and sometimes via games, especially among young people.

Humanity has advanced as a result of people's approach to others with a sense of sharing. The oldest instinct of human, moreover, is that which impels him/her to get in contact with others. The end state of not having any kind of relationship with others is seen among the mentally handicapped (Adler, 2017b: 289–293). Individuals' forming a society is possible with socializing. And forming a society is possible with communication. An individual, expresses himself/herself, produces ideas and improves himself/herself by sharing with others (Akyazı ve Akyazı, 2013: 206). Rapid advancement of the communication media and society's interest and demand on these have brought a new dimension to the term "socializing" (Akyazı, 2015: 175).

Player's *habitus* on virtual space defines his/her transition between real life and virtual space and social relations with other players. Player's fighting or uniting forces or coming together to create specific rules and spaces against a common goal has caused "a new type of tribalism" to come to exist… Players come together and play games, enter into social relations and express themselves with a sense of belonging imagined and made real in virtual space similar to a nation's being an imagined community (Binark ve Sütçü, 2008: 54).

People have two worlds today. One is the natural one. Flesh and blood, this world is the place where the humanity has existed since Homo Sapiens. People build up countless relationships with others face to face. They create social patterns, laws and education systems, and codes of conduct. Moreover, they are influenced by the instinct formed by countless encounters with other people. According to Bagdikian, the other world in which most of the humanity live is the world in mass media. The changes in this period, dating back as old as Gutenberg's invention of printing press, have finally altered traditional kingdoms and social religious orders of the ages. Modern mass media in industrialized nations has changed social relationships, politics, economy and legal structures. Most of the individuals of industrialized nations spend most of their time in this new world (Bagdikian, 2004: 13). Thanks to the effort to pass on everything happening in real life to this new world, people find their way into this world via countless information, entertainment and activities.

While information is the most important notion defining our age, getting caught up in this information and not being able to catch up with it is also a handicap of our age. "Ignorance has three types: Not knowing what is necessary, knowing the one of poor quality and knowing the unnecessary" (Topçu, as cited in Girgin ve Erkal, 2018: 151). These are the type of situations we are encountering these days. Along with the new media, information is pouring on us instantly, with no delay. Since we receive information on something instantly, as soon as we receive further information the old one becomes invalid and outdated. In the world of electrical shaping, we are in a position to abandon our habit of data classification and to adopt a pattern of recognition as a pattern (McLuhan ve Fiore, 2005: 63). With our age's technology, we are exposed to so much information that we often have information about subjects that we are not interested in or that we do not need. Thanks to the machines that change our perception, learning skills and style, we can neither do business nor spend time without them.

Instead of becoming the master of the machines human created, she/he has become their servant. However, human beings are not created to be objectified. Despite the saturation provided by the consumption, the powers that the human possesses cannot be left in constant uncertainty. According to Fromm, we have only one choice, that is, to regain the management of the machines, to use it in the name of man's development by making a means rather than an end of production. Otherwise, the digested life energies will reveal themselves in a complex and destructive way. Instead of dying in distress, one will have to destroy life (Fromm, 2001: 81). At first, we used social media as a leisure activity and to get rid of our troubles; over time we have had to work for it with a great effort. People of this new world called "Social Media Slaves" also consume a great part of their lives in these circles.

According to Andreas Kaplan and Michael Haenlein, social media is a group of internet-based applications built on ideological and technological bases that allow users to make changes or interact with new individuals. A significant increase in the use of social media in recent years has changed both individual and corporate communication. The rapid change of social media allows users to connect with people they do not know and think more openly and quickly (Altunbaş, 2014: 9–10).

Speaking of socializing not only with the people they did not know, but even with the machine and saying "Welcome to the era of social machines" Semmelhack refers to any type of machine or tool or an object connected to the internet as a social connection. In this world called internet of things, next thing you know your fridge has started to follow you on Twitter, and you are friends on Facebook with your brother's car (Semmelhack, 2013: 6). It can be said that a world as in an episode of the Black Mirror where a woman maintains her relationship with a computer that acts like her dead husband by mimicking the characteristics of him via the information on his social media accounts is not far away.

Machines that can perform cognitive tasks are more important than machines capable of performing physical tasks. Thanks to modern artificial intelligence, it is now possible to produce these machines. Our digital machines have begun to break down chains that restrict themselves and recognize patterns and communicate complexly and show skills on other areas which were once only in our monopoly (Brynjolfsson ve McAfee, 2015: 109). The virtual reality and the augmented reality technologies that draw attention with the fantasies that they produce are developing and spreading day by day.

Virtual reality is a term for computer-generated 3D environments that make people feel like they are living in the environment they see. Users are involved in virtual environments/worlds through a variety of peripherals (such as a helmet-mounted display). From that moment onwards, the user is disconnected from reality and experiences the feeling of being in the environment in which the virtual reality is created. The virtual reality environments vary according to the intensity (level) of the reality sentiment that the participant creates (Sanal Gerçeklik (VR) Nedir?, n.d.).

In virtual reality technology, the user looks at the screen where the individual creates a three-dimensional perception by combining two images, designed for each eye, rather than looking at a flat screen. The screen used in virtual reality technology is displayed at a frame rate of 90 to 120 frames per second. This speed is a speed that is necessary for the human brain to perceive a visual as if it was a reality. Such a high level of speed allows the user to be fully engaged in adapting to the virtual real world (Yengin ve Bayrak, 2017: 106). So, it takes a certain time for the person who spent a long time in the virtual reality environment to get out of the simulation and get back to the real world.

The discovery of optical signals is an important part of the development process of virtual reality technology. With optical signals, the system calculates the position information of the individual and positions the object in the digital environment. At the same time, the system provides the follow-up of the object by measuring the distance between the sensors and the object. This measurement continues as long as the system is running (Yengin ve Bayrak, 2018: 48). Individuals who are provided with physical freedom of movement with some additional devices and detectors can also have a near-real life experience.

The simulation is trying to eliminate the absence of the real phenomenon and to create a reality effect in this sense. In fact, real and fake are contradictory concepts, and they cannot replace each other. However, the simulation is increasing its effectiveness day by day in an effort to remove this distinction. In a virtual world, a person who experiences a pre-designed and coded data as if it was reality can also get the chance to be in an environment that cannot be found in real life (Yengin ve Bayrak, 2017: 87, 117). At the same time, he/she can create an escapist fantasy space by resorting to the simulation to escape from situations he/she does not want to be in real life. By entering the simulation universe, the person who is moving away from the reality and the real life has the desire to return over and over again to the satisfaction he/she attains here.

Escapist Fantasy

Interaction of modern human beings with their external reality is not by direct means. Especially in his/her communications, which are so extensive as to conceive a way of life, sees, evaluates, and makes sense of the external reality through the types of mass communication that describe this external reality on his/her behalf. For example, in the cinema, the audience becomes Immortal Gods. While watching the characters who live their own limited lives in cinema, the audience is alive at the end of everything. Thus, the cinema makes the audience feel immortal. This delusion (the fantasy of being able to stay alive after everything is done) relieves the audience in a contemporary society that is rapidly changing and where the moment everything is formed fully, death happens (Oskay, 1994: 60).

We are inevitably looking for remedies in the world of fiction, literature and theater for what we lost in life. There we find people who know how to die, even those who have managed to kill someone else. We can only find possible condition – that is, the condition that we must be able to protect life as it is despite the rise and fall – that we can compromise with death (Freud, 2007a: 77).

Fantasy has functioned in the lightening of the shock created by the new or unexpected in the living period (Oskay, 1994: 57). Fantasia is an aesthetic perception which continuously surpasses the boundaries of real and normal states and understandings. Fantasy may be a desire for change and the idea of realizing what we have in mind or what things have implied to us (Hume, as cited in Yılmaz, 2010: 4).

Fantasy is not real. It is a kind of activity that does not obligate to solve problems and to act for purpose. For example, viewing violence in a fantasy setting reduces spiritual tension. Fantasy canalizes aggression to substitution target instead of real target. It enables hostility and fragility to be revealed harmlessly. Thus, one experiences catharsis. The view that plain violence does not lead the audience to violence is defended by the hypothesis of catharsis (as cited in Yengin, 1997: 162).

"Catharsis" is the job of getting rid of distressing emotions by expressing them. While tragedy as an archaic ritual provides catharsis, it is said that violent publications of today fulfill this mission. The fear and horror we witness virtually in detail are said to purify our soul from passion. The concept of catharsis used by Aristotle for the first time means that the tragedia acts as a purifier for the unhappiness of the audience. The essence of catharsis is to discharge stress, tension, in an expressible form (as cited in Yengin, 1997: 162). The function that tragedies have once made is now provided by new media even interactively and more actively. With digital games, the person who takes on the character he/she wants can destroy everything and everyone he/she does not want. Particularly during periods of adolescence and in case of anger and insufficiency against collective or life-threatening situations, violence-related games can be used to discharge purify. The only feeling that needs to be discharged is not the feeling of violence. In terms of psychoanalysis, other important emotions and instincts must also be fulfilled.

The feeling of weakness or "inferiority" is the root concept of individual psychology (Adler, 2016: 73). Disability is a positive pain and at least continues as long as the task is not completed, the need is not addressed or a tension does not end. It is an emotion that is obviously from nature. It is like a painful tension that one wants to get rid of. According to Freud, this liberation or relaxation does not have to be pleasing, but it can bring a feeling of liking (Adler, 2017c: 82). The inability to solve the three basic problems of life (society, profession and, love) in a timely manner or to prepare for it requires, produces an inferiority complex in the individual, and an unsuccessful balance of it produces superiority complex (Adler, 2018: 9). New media users who want to satisfy this superiority complex in everyday life either provide it with digital games they have succeeded (with the points they have earned and the feeling of winning), or they are satisfied with the enjoyment they receive through the superior and perfect worlds they have established in virtual worlds.

According to Adler, sexual instinct has a place in the power that pushes the person to be successful and superior, but this desire and effort to be superior is the most effective factor in creating human personality. Adler does not entirely deny the importance of sexual instinct, which holds a crucial place in Freud's psychology, but claims that this instinct has no such a big importance and role in human life as Freud says. According to Adler, this driving force is what life calls positive strength; "Creative self" is the same thing. The individual is a creature who has to give effort to be superior and to give a speed and direction to his life by trying to be superior when he/she has any sense of inferiority. An individual is also disturbed by an organic or psychological disorder or a feeling of inadequacy due to deficiency. This inferiority that conflicts with the desire to be superior turns into a disturbing factor, often unconscious feeling called inferiority complex, when not properly canalized. In this respect, the individual will try to convince himself and others of this by believing that the influence of this sensation is either achieving or succeeding (Adler, 2017a: 76).

People have social and psychological needs. As a result of these needs, people will enter into anticipation to get their needs out of the media and other sources. According to the Uses and Gratifications approach, which is based on Katz's research and work, viewers use media content to meet a number of needs. As a result of this usage, the audience needs to be satisfied, that is, the needs are satisfied, and therefore the audience gets satisfied using the media contents towards their needs. They expose some of these needs in the context of exposure to the media. However, there may also be some unwanted or unintended consequences as the media effect (Yaylagül, 2006: 62).

Modernity, which stigmatizes and at the same time compensates for the durability and impasse of everyday life, cannot deprive itself of adventure passion. However, "bureaucratically guided consumption society" drowned this passion in repetitive routines and stereotyped values and practices – certainly the societies living between the indicators of consumption (Köse, 2008: 10). When we look into the modern world, we are confronted with a generation that is constantly directed to consuming and shopping malls as free time activity. It is tried to attain a sense of superiority by consuming more and owing more expensive things in today's consumer societies. Using the latest technology products or having expensive tastes and showing them to people through social media is aimed at satisfying this feeling.

The everydayness, as Lefebvre says, is seen as "an escape area encouraged by an ideological mass culture". On the other hand, the reproduction of everyday life takes place intensively through sedentary media. Lefebvre sees sedentary media which accompanies link of relations combining an alienating everyday with the act of consuming as the end of an idealistic political structure. (...) In Lefebvrian way of thinking which precedes Baudrillard, the argument "constant one dimensionality will be disrupted sooner or later as to give way to dreams and new fantasias" presented as the only escape from overwhelming - at the same time productive – atmosphere of everyday is also inspired by the upending continuity of the same system (Köse, 2008: 10).

George Ritzer and Chris Rojek say that leisure, recreation and consumerism are in fact the address of escapist trends and serve to escape the rationality of our lives (Aytaç, 2006: 46). Cultural industries vulgarize aesthetic arts and turn enjoyment into distraction or entertainment. Thus, it paves the way to the entertainment society. Although entertainment serves to escape the rationality of life, this escape route in fact is towards a world that is again rational and bureaucratic. Dispersed from one escape to the other, the individual's route is directed to fantasy and hyperreality (Aytaç, 2004:127). The method to achieve pleasure is also the universe of simulations which make fantasies and dreams that come true.

There is a strong tendency towards the principle of pleasure in the soul, but this conflicts with other powers or relationships, and the result may not always be in accordance with the principle of pleasure (Freud, 2016b: 23). It is now easier to fulfill dreams, desires and wishes in the state of digital ecstasy that we reach through virtual drugs to get pleasure.

The functions of dreams have also been the fulfillment of the wish in a delusional way under the rule of the pleasure principle (Freud, 2000: 217). However, this relaxation and unloader treatment through dreams that cannot be controlled is always now accessible and controllable with state of ecstasy, thanks to digital methods. Thanks to the new technologies, more and more realistic dreams have been created and the doors of unlimited satisfaction have been opened.

Digital Ecstasy

Digital ecstasy refers to an ecstasy, numbness due to the simulation and fantasies created with advanced technologies. The concept of technological dream (Övür, 2009: 90) refers to the fantasies created in the digital environment, while the digital ecstatic state refers to the feeling and the situation felt by them under their influence. Even though it has a temporary impact such as detachment from the world, the inability to perceive reality, and the alienation from life and environment; the amount of time spent in the case of digital ecstasy increases day by day due to its pleasure and satisfaction.

The time it takes to return to real life and the time it takes for the perceptions to reach the right judgments on reality vary according to the digital environment and time. For example, the difference and effect of a person connecting to a digital environment using virtual reality to watch television and enter the fantasy world will be of different dimensions. The degree of satisfaction experienced due to the sense of reality will also increase.

The common features of the researches based on the Uses and Gratifications approach are that people have social and psychological needs and act on the premise that they are searching for media content to satisfy these needs. People can meet their needs by consuming certain media contents. Studies based on this approach, on the contrary to the tradition of more deterministic impact research, focus on the capacity of individuals to search, find and use media contents consciously and voluntarily according to their needs and desires (Yaylagül, 2006: 62). According to Rosengren, for people to take action, needs should emerge as a problem. Rosengren therefore focuses on the biological and psychological infrastructure that underlie human behavior. People react by acting on these two bases. The basic needs of human beings include: 1) psychological needs, 2) security needs, 3) needs of belonging and love, 4) reputation needs and 5) self-realization needs (Ayhan ve Çavuş, 2014: 38).

In communication studies, communication processes, institutional structures and communication systems are never separated from the social, economic, political and cultural structures in which communication systems are formed and developed (Yaylagül, 2006: 21). Each of these structures determines the extent to which we use the media, and the media we use undoubtedly affect these structures. When we look at Turkey today, it is seen that there are cultural, political and economic obstacles in meeting people's social and psychological need. Today, people are trying the virtual world in order to set up an effective and satisfying relationship with the opposite sex in Turkey which has the traces of religious and conservative history when people were prevented from contacting with each other. Once women who got the message across the men they liked by dropping their handkerchiefs are doing it with *likes* and via social media now. While expressing their political ideas (especially to avoid the potential problems of expressing the contrary ones), the abstaining people prefer new media environments in order to satisfy these feelings by reading and watching others. From an economic point of view, people who are from a low income group who know that the money in their pocket will decrease every time they decide to leave the house and go to a place, they see new media environments which offer many alternatives as leisure activities. The fact that the habit of reading books at home is almost absent and the habit of watching television decreases among young people by turning to new media, watching the series from the Internet without interruption, making smart phones widespread, the development of internet connections and their becoming cheaper make the virtual world become a center of attraction.

There are many different psychological reasons for people to turn to virtual media and fantasies. In general, the average person gets the feeling of insecurity, loneliness and oppression; and in the middle of the abundance, he satisfies with a handful of pleasure. Life does not mean anything to him; he is aware that he cannot make any sense to life as a consumer and being nothing after all. One could not withstand the meaninglessness and self-indulgence of life if the system did not offer a wide range of television (and internet) broadcasts that would allow him/her the opportunity to move away from the facts in order not to realize that he/she had lost more of its values every day (Fromm, 2001: 80).

For example, if a society cannot feed most or a large part of its members sufficiently, they must satisfy them with a diseased narcissism in order to prevent social unrest. For people who are economically and culturally poor, the narcissistic pride of being a member of that community is one – and often very effective – a source of satisfaction. These people can develop an extreme narcissism because their life does not bring something interesting to them and does not provide the opportunity to improve their interest (Fromm, 1994: 71). It also nourishes and keeps narcissism fresh continuously through the media.

The personality line is always on the move, and as if all the senses associated with our personal situation sometimes create a slight sense of restlessness and insecurity, a correction tends to support and exalt the life (Adler, 2015: 72). The person says that I am also here through the social media channel and the individual who is trying to "harmonize" with such expressions "I am the best, beautiful, perfect, I love myself" in line with the 'effort of making us compatible with the society, in which we live is included in the social media channel and the narcissistic aspect of the person emerges through the means in this field. In general, social media includes the dynamics that encourage narcissism in terms of tools and environment (Alanka and Cezik, 2016: 560). It also fulfills the function of satisfying this narcissism. The person is seeking happiness by exposing his/her perfect world, which is not very similar to the reality created by virtual media.

According to the Uses and Gratifications approach, the media is the source that enables the audience to meet their own needs. The audience uses this resource rationally according to their needs. According to this, the viewers can interpret the broadcasts in a very different way and can produce conclusions apart from the given message. This approach highlights the audience's own logic and subjectivity (Yaylagül, 2006: 63). In the context of the uses and gratifications approach, the new virtual reality applications, with the developing technology and the internet, have now enabled the user to choose from more options and have begun to watch his choice not to be imposed on him. The limited number of options on television has reached the infinite number with the internet. Therefore, users have the chance to reach as much as gratification they want at any time. These fantasies, which have the effect of discharging, just like in dreams, have paved the way for an indispensable and manageable dream world for users.

Dreams are fantasies like modern fantasies that have effects of catharsis and discharging treatment which our world of imagination, what we live, what we want to live, what we have to suppress because we cannot live and our subconscious have revealed. It is not possible to select and control dreams, but it is in our hands to control and select the virtual reality and simulation fantasies that we can see as a kind of technological dream that provides a similar purification with dreams. These fantasies provide a similar purification and help us discharge. When we examine the concept of dream with this approach, we bear in mind that we are also examining the concept of virtual reality.

Dreams are an effort to find solutions to the problems faced by individuals in an easy way. The function of dreams is to stand to the challenges facing us and solve them. The difficulties come lighter than they are in the dream, and the solution offered in the dream does not expect us to make much effort. What is the purpose of dream? A psychoanalyst responds to the question why we dream by saying "to satisfy the unfulfilled wishes". The Greeks and the Egyptians spent nights in the temples expecting to be rewarded with a sacred dream that might affect their future life; they believed that the dreams seen there had ameliorated and alleviated physical and mental illness (Adler, 2017b: 108–114).

According to Burdach, the purpose of dreams is to save us from everyday life. Even when our mind is fully filled with a matter, we are deeply troubled, or our mental power is engaged with a problem, the dream does nothing but enter our soul and express the reality with symbols. Fichte, in the same sense, actually speaks of "complementary dreams" and defines them as one of the hidden blessings of the soul's self-healing nature (as cited in Freud, 2016c: 66).

Freud sees dreams as reflections of unconscious desires. In the dream, as in neurotic disorders and unintentional forgetfulness, our desires that we do not want to appear and therefore pushed out of our consciousness, show themselves as having changed their form (Fromm, 2003: 69). In every dream, an instinctive desire must be expressed as realized and saturated. The breakdown of the spiritual life from the reality at night and the regression to the primitive mechanisms that make it possible allow the desired instinctual satisfaction to be experienced in an illusionary way as if it were happening now (Freud, 2007b: 45). This feeling "as if it is happening now" is a satisfying feature that we also feel in virtual reality. In virtual reality, we turn to the fantasies like dreams in line with the wishes and desires of our subconscious. When we look at the most watched series on the Internet, it is seen that all over the world, series such as Game of Thrones (GoT) which uncovers the myths, instincts and repressive impulses (death, sexuality, incest, murder, violence and destruction) lead the way.

Freud sees the dream analysis as via regia (royal highway) going to the direction of the out-of-consciousness route. It goes directly to the deepest personal secrets, so it is an invaluable tool in the hands of the psychologist and the instructor (Jung, 2016b: 37). Dream is also a creative act. Even the average people recognize and realize their creative aspects that they never realized when they are awake in dream. One of the facts revealed by Freud is the existence of censorship in the dream. Dreams should not only be understood as the unconscious motives becoming conscious. Censorship that appears in the dream changes the true meaning of the dream. This phenomenon of censorship, which is located behind a curtain, allows the hidden thoughts to cover the boundaries of consciousness only when they are adequately covered and masked (Fromm, 2004b: 112).

After his detailed research on dreams, Freud made remarkable distinctions between the conscious and unconscious aspects of the soul. It was revealed that no organization or coordination other than consciousness was involved, and that each tendency pursued the pursuit of satisfaction independently of the others, and that the tendencies that worked against each other could stand side by side. Thus, the connotations of ideas other than consciousness continue their way without considering the logical contexts (Freud, 2016a: 17). According to Jung, the unconscious is a psychological border line concept in psychology, which includes all psychic contents or processes that are not consciously meaningless to a relationship with the ego (Jung, 2016c: 14). Jung says that in the analysis of the personal subconscious, the first thing to be added to consciousness is the personal content, and that these unconscious contents, which may be repressed, but which can come to consciousness, should be given the name of the personal unconscious (Jung, 2016b: 179).

According to Freud, satisfying all instinctual wishes unhindered will create mental health and happiness (Fromm, 2007: 106). As a result, it was revealed that all of the unconscious contents of the soul, such as the longings and desires, consisted of the tendencies determined through will, and that they provided their energies directly from basic physical impulses. The only goal they want to achieve directly is absolute satisfaction and they can often fall from the diameter through the conscious elements of the spirit world, which is necessary to confront and adapt to the reality and to protect against external threats (Freud, 2017c, 16). However, the suppressed urge never stops trying to achieve full satisfaction by insisting on the repetition of a primary satisfaction life (Freud, 2016b: 51).

If man could really shake his unconscious, he could suck its energy and immobilize it, it would be a perfect solution. But experiences show that the energy of the unconscious can only be partially destroyed: the unconscious is in constant activity, because it contains not only libido, but also its source (Jung, 2016b: 191).

It is certainly true that unconscious desires remain active. These represent the paths that can always be passed when a certain amount of stimulation is available. Indeed, indestructibility is a predominant feature of unconscious processes. Nothing out of consciousness can be terminated, nothing can stay in the past or be unforgettable. This is most evident when examining neuroses and hysteria. The unconscious thought pathway that causes the hysteresis to discharge immediately becomes repetitive when adequate stimulation accumulates (Freud, 2016d: 359). The ideas that the psychological behaviors that seem to be randomized are determined precisely contribute to good results in psychology, and perhaps in law, for a very long time. Bleuler and Jung were able to make sense of the behavior obtained in their experiments called "association" (Freud, 2014: 277).

According to the theory that Jung has gathered under the name of "analytical psychology", each person has an external and inner world. According to Jung, there is an energetic structure called "entity" such as the magma layer at the center of the globe, which appears to be the essence of our inner self, which can be considered as the essence of our inner self. At the top, we defined the "persona" for our environment and the characteristics we gained as a result of the harmony to the environment and culture we live in. If we adopt the social pattern without questioning it with our own brains, blindly, we may lose our relationship with our personality. This structure of ours which Jung calls "shadow personality" consists of intellectual and actional approaches that happen when our consciousness is freed from pressure, which can be observed in alcohol users that we cannot recognize (Adler, 2017d: 40–41). This structure, called a shadow personality, is also a factor that affects the choices of people by appearing in the case of digital ecstasy and constantly seeks satisfaction.

While the reasons that lead to digital ecstasy are similar to alcohol, alcoholic drunkenness is only a relief and perhaps there is an effect such as forgetting those requests, but in digital ecstasy these are realized and satisfied at least in virtual life. This is exactly the same as in a psychoanalytic study and has the effect of neutralizing them by talking rather than hiding the emotions or covering them. It can be described as relaxation by releasing the pressed energy as in Freud's treatment of the hysteria (initially hypnosis and then the method of free association). Here we have an emptying treatment by identifying our free associations with our free choices and not in the presence of a psychiatrist. For example, a teenager angry at life and his surrounding is looking for relaxation by turning towards violent games in a world that is under his control. Or you cannot always see the person you are in love in person, yet you can watch them constantly on the internet and meet this desire object somehow. By this, you are fortunate enough to join their life and experiences by looking and liking their photos.

According to Freud, it is interesting to note that although the number of survival opportunities as a single person is limited, it is interesting to note that the civilization's self-sacrifice is felt as an overwhelming burden by the civilization in order to live together with others (Freud, 2017a: 28). Human beings have to adapt to two fronts; first, the external life – to the profession, family, society – and secondly to the vital demands of its nature. Neglecting any of these demands leads to illness. Some people are neurotic because of external causes, others for internal reasons (Jung, 2016a: 110). Neurosis is, according to Adler, a distorted form of adaptation to deceive oneself and those around them rather than face the truth and do what is necessary. By adopting a neurotic behavior, the individual thinks that there is a way of adapting to himself. However, the sense of satisfaction that the individual has in this evasive way is costly and makes him/her abnormal (Adler, 2017a: 77). As neurologists have found various solutions to forget the problematic issue, today people see fantasies as a solution to escape from the truth and to get away.

Illusions look good to us because it protects us from pain and allows us to enjoy. Therefore, we must accept that without any complaint; the illusions will be broken into pieces when they collide with reality (Freud, 2017b: 66). Although the illusions offered by the technology provide us with pleasure and satisfaction, the problems caused by the excessive and unconscious use of the virtual world should not be ignored. Especially young people can easily share because they are not very knowledgeable about the possibilities of being blacklisted or having negative results. He/she can share everything even the things that in real life he/she hides or never talks to anyone from his/her sexual choices to political thoughts. However, middle-aged and older users of virtual worlds are more aware of the fact that these channels are a part of real life and they are more careful. Thinking of being a part of the surveillance they re-think 10 times about sharing while it is the opposite case in young people. In conjunction with digital technologies, surveillance has become an inevitable problem, sometimes even paranoia. Are they spying on me from the camera on my computer or phone? Are the things I say over the phone (or when my smartphone is with me) stored and saved? Questions like many have begun to pass through. Those who put black bands on their computer's camcorder or who pay attention to their calls and searches are increasing.

Everyday life is confronted with the process of social media, the political system, the economy, the expansion and intensification of surveillance. Surveillance means managing the population and controlling an individual's behavior (Çakır, 2014: 128). According to Fuchs, surveillance is instrumental and is a tool used to try and benefit certain groups or individuals to the detriment of other groups and individuals. Surveillance is based on competition. It tries to protect or carry out certain behaviors of groups or individuals through the collection, storage, processing, dissemination, evaluation and use of data about people. Thus, potential or actual physical, ideological or structural violence can be directed towards people in order to influence people's behavior. This effect is carried out by the means of repression and provides benefits to specific groups to the detriment of others (Fuchs, 2014: 218).

For example, while we spend many hours on Facebook and watch the lives of others; Facebook is watching and storing our lives, ideologies, tastes, things we love, loved ones and things we do unconsciously. After the discovery of this information was used during the last presidential election in the USA, Facebook has experienced hard times and is trying to recover its lost reputation. This information can be used to serve all purposes – from which candidate we will vote for, which product we will consume and whom we will marry.

That fake takes the place of the truth and the truth is fictionalized into false is a situation we encounter a lot today. In terms of pushing the boundaries of imitating the real life, the virtual world and its applications are now surpassing the real life and put its eyes on fate which is luck according to some or divine power to the others. Facebook's latest work also reflects this. The following example may be more illustrative: one day a doctor who had been in the same places (Mexico, Cuba) as I had been and taken pictures from similar angles sent me a friend request and I accepted thinking that we had met in one of these places. But when I asked, he said that we had never met before and had added me through Facebook's recommendations section. Why would Facebook have suggested me to someone who does not even have one common friend, but is a lot like me? Was that one of our paranoia we experience? Or data mining? In his profile it also wrote doctor like mine. How many people could there be – from the opposite sex who are both doctor in Turkey and have been to those both countries and taken photos at the same angle? (It was almost like he was photoshopped into my photos.) When I thought that there would not be too many people, I thought that this match was deliberate. Just as I asked people around me to tell me if they experience anything like this, few days later one of my friends told me that Mark Zuckerberg – the founder of Facebook – had announced that such application would be initiated. News ("Facebook çöpçatanlık uygulaması başlatıyor", 2018) said that, Facebook's matchmaking application will begin to test and people with similar tastes and features will be matched with each other and appear in the recommendations section. In particular, Zuckerberg proudly explained that they are working for a long-term relationship model that was different from other similar applications. Facebook is now refreshing both the image and aiming to re-awaken the decreasing attention of the youth. Knowing that this technology is possible confirms the idea of the new divine power, which states that our fate is in the hands of digital technologies. And it is a new element that will connect people to the virtual world a little more.

The simulation is about to win the war with reality. It seems that this struggle will continue until there are no real cases left in the real world that cannot be moved to the virtual world. Maybe we can build a country called Digitalia in the virtual world and make the whole world its citizens. There everyone can have a body of their wish and behave freely. They can choose both physical and personality characteristics as they wish. At certain intervals, a chairman is elected and takes over the government by the election held among Digitalia citizens. In this Digitopia, people can realize all their desires and wishes they want to do in real life. They can go into an eternal digital ecstasy and survive in a virtual life like in an Avatar. Who can claim that dreams do not turn into reality someday?

We teach our children that we are more advanced than the generations before us and that there is nothing that has not been realized, nothing that cannot be achieved. The result supports this idea, which is etched into our brain without stopping (Fromm, 2006: 15). Man would have been the lord of the machines he created, but he has been its butler. However, man is not created to become an object. Nevertheless, despite all the slogans, we are rapidly adapting to the society governed by bureaucrats who manage a well-fed, cared, inhumane, oppressed mass man. "We manufacture machined people and humanized machines". Fifty years ago, this was one of the biggest criticisms of socialism. Thus, this would lead to bureaucratization, sameness, centralization and soulless materialism, whereas these are the realities of today's capitalism. We are talking about freedom and democracy, but a growing number of people fear of having the responsibility of freedom and favor the captivity of a well-fed robot (Fromm, 2001: 80–81). We are faced with a community of people living in a real virtuality and a "social media slavery". Looking at the monotonous robotic faces that are similar to each other, we look for the truth, but we cannot find it. We are in the era of people who live in a real virtuality, people who apply botox to look young, use social media to look social and use fake smiles to look happy. Virtual reality and real virtuality is the reality of our times...

Of course, among innumerable changes in nature, individuals who have better opportunities, can find the best shape, and thus fit in the best manner in the environment, have a better chance of success (Adler, 2017d: 165). With the awareness that technology is the most important fact of our time, we try to adapt to every technological development and innovation but when we look at what they make us lose, the success of technology is shadowed.

Human behavior is goal-oriented and interactive. All individuals and societies are holistic, and the individual gains importance in the social system according to their behavior. (Adler, 2017d: 43). According to Fromm, "Sociology only embraces society and psychology only embraces the individual" is wrong. Because psychology deals with the socialized individual and sociology deals with a group of individuals whose mental structure and mechanisms need to be taken into consideration (Fromm, 2004a: 58). Psychoanalysis has been able to show that people's ideologies are a product of instinctive impulses, interests, needs and expressing themselves as largely unconsciously rationalizing. Psychoanalysis has evolved on the basis of instinctual impulses and biologically defined instincts, and their quantitative and content are influenced by the individual's socioeconomic status or class (Fromm, 2005: 179).

According to Adler, man is a conscious animal who is aware of his acts. With self-study, he can find out why he's acting like this. Consciousness is the essence of the person. A person is aware of what he does every day. According to him, this does not mean denying what he does unconsciously; to give the right to the conscious (Adler, 2017a: 65). When people become aware of what they are doing, it becomes easier to control their movements. However, as there is a resistance in every patient during psychoanalysis, it can also be misleading or rejection in the way people understand and analyze what they are doing and can be lost within illusions by deceiving themselves.

Conclusion

Throughout the ages, mankind has used a variety of methods to go beyond reality or to cope with reality. Parallel to his/her world of imagination; with illusions, pretending, dreams and fantasies, he/she has escaped from the facts that he/she did not want to be real and approached to the ones that he/she wants to be real. With the introduction of the media into human life by technology, day-by-day fantasies are more accessible, used and competed with realities.

Due to the simulations and fantasies created with advanced technologies; the time spent during digital ecstasy which refers to the divergence from reality, blackout and numbness has increased every day. There are significant differences between the digital ecstasy in the radio days where the first developments in the field of media were achieved, and the digital ecstasy in the worlds created by today's new media and virtual reality technologies.

Thanks to the development of the internet, people can easily reach saturation by using programs and applications that are suitable for their needs. Thus, with catharsis and discharging treatment, they can reach happiness in their lives for a short time at least. Although the digital fields turned to with the desire and the need to have this happiness last are not successful at providing the same satisfaction every time, once a person is kept happy, he/she is repeatedly connected to the digital media with the hope of getting the same satisfaction again. Are virtual reality fantasies like dreams in terms of their effects on people, reflecting our subconscious, personality, what we suppress, and what we have covered? Are people intentionally or unintentionally looking for such fantasies? are some questions to be considered.

Our suppressed and covered feelings which need saturating yet cannot be saturated because of social oppression and cultural imperatives make us turn to virtual environments more. We experience things that cannot be experienced in real life or would be penalized in virtual world and create ourselves fields of relief. Instead of experiencing life, we look for and find satisfaction with virtual sedatives. We experience love, violence, goodness, evil, tension and happiness in the virtual reality and get so saturated that we do not need for the real ones. As in tragedies once, we are watching the problems and big issues of others in the dramas, and sometimes we shed a tear and relax thinking our problems are only the small ones. Sometimes we find peace seeing similar problems and feeling "it's not just me".

Our biggest fears are confronted in a safe environment. The release of fear is liberating man, but it feels good to be still alive. Since the gratifications acquired in digital media appeal to both eye and ear and also emotions, they create almost the same effect as the reality once enough concentration is provided. However, it differs from the reality in that the happiness and gratification last for a short time. Realizing it is unreal, and having it back on consciousness, one, again, experiences dissatisfaction. For this happiness to last, we should either be in virtual world all the time or strong enough to face the reality and became aware.

Bibliography

Adler, A. (2015). Bireysel Psikoloji (A. Kılıçoğlu, Trans.). İstanbul: Say Yayınları.

Adler, A. (2016). Nevroz Sorunları (A. Kılıçoğlu, Trans.). İstanbul: Say Yayınları.

Adler, A. (2017a). Sosyal Roller ve Kişilik (T. Yörükan, Trans.). İstanbul: Türkiye İş Bankası Kültür Yayınları.

Adler, A. (2017b). Yaşamın Anlam ve Amacı (K. Şipal, Trans.). İstanbul: Say Yayınları.

Adler, A. (2017c). Yaşama Sanatı (E. Günsel, Trans.). Ankara: Tutku Yayınevi.

Adler, A. (2017d). Modern Psikoloji (M. Uhrayoğlu, Trans.). Ankara: Yason Yayınları.

Adler, A. (2018). Sorunlu Okul Çocuğu (K. Şipal, Trans.). İstanbul: Say Yayınları.

Akyazı, A. (2015). Gazetelerin Haber Paylaşım Platformu olarak sosyal medyanın çatışma kültürüne etkisi. In T. Kara & E. Özgen (Eds.), Ağdaki Şüphe Bir Sosyal Medya Eleştirisi (pp. 171–190). İstanbul: Beta Yayınları.

Akyazı, E. & Akyazı, A. (2013). Yeni Bir Demokrasi Plaftormu Olarak Sosyal Medya: TBMM 24. Dönem Milletvekillerinin "Twitter" Ortamındaki Mevcudiyetleri ve "Suriye Krizi" Üzerinden Mesaj İçeriklerinin Analizi. In A. Algül & N. Üçer (Eds.), Yeni Medya'da Demokrasi (pp. 205–225). İstanbul: Literatürk Yayınları.

Alanka, Ö. & Cezik, A. (2016). Dijital Kibir: Sosyal Medyadaki Narsistik Ritüellere İlişkin Bir İnceleme. TRT akademi, 1(2), 549–569.

Altunbaş, F. (2014). Sosyal Medyanın Gücü. Konya: Çizgi Kitabevi.

Ayhan, B. & Çavuş, S. (2014). İzleyici Araştırmalarında Değişim: Kullanımlar ve Doyumlardan Bağımlılığa. Selçuk İletişim, 8(2), 32–60.

Aytaç, Ö. (2004). Kapitalizm ve Hegemonya İlişkileri Bağlamında Serbest Zaman. C.Ü. Sosyal Bilimler Dergisi, 28(2), 115–138.

Aytaç, Ö. (2006). Tüketimcilik ve Metalaşma Kıskacında Boş Zaman. Kocaeli Üniversitesi Sosyal Bilimler Enstitüsü Dergisi, 2006/1(11), 27–53.

Bagdikian B. H. (2004). Yeni Medya Tekeli (E. Eminel, Trans.). Ankara: Akılçelen Kitaplar.

Binark, M. & Sütçü, B. G. (2008). Dijital Oyun. İstanbul: Kalkedon Yayınları.

Brynjolfsson, E. & McAfee, A. (2015). The Second Machine Age. Akıllı Teknolojiler Devrinde Çalışma, İlerleme ve Refah (E. Eminel, Trans.). İstanbul: Türk Hava Yolları Yayınları.

Çakır, M. (2014). Yeni Medyaya İlişkin Eleştirel Yaklaşımları ve Tespitleri ile Christian Fuchs. In M. Çakır (Ed.), Yeni Medyaya Eleştirel Yaklaşımlar (pp. 81–130). İstanbul: Doğu Kitapevi.

Facebook çöpçatanlık uygulaması başlatıyor. (2018, May 2). CNNTürk. Retrieved from https://www.cnnturk.com/video/dunya/facebook-copcatanlik-uygulamasi-baslatiyor. on 4 May 2018.

Freud, S. (2000). Metapsikoloji (A. Yardımlı, Trans.). İstanbul: İdea Yayınevi.

Freud, S. (2007a). Uygarlık, Din ve Toplum (S. Budak, Trans.). İstanbul: Öteki Yayınevi.

Freud, S. (2007b). Psikanalize Yeni Giriş Dersleri (S. Budak, Trans.). İstanbul: Öteki Yayınevi.

Freud, S. (2014). Günlük Yaşamın Psikopatolojisi (H. Can, Trans.). Ankara: Tutku Yayınevi.

Freud, S. (2016a). Nevrozlar (K. Şipal, Trans.). İstanbul: Say Yayınları.

Freud, S. (2016b). Haz İlkesinin Ötesinde Ben ve İd (S. Babaoğlu, Trans.). İstanbul: Metis Yayınları.

Freud, S. (2016c). Rüyaların Yorumu (S. Budak, Trans.). İstanbul: Öteki Yayınevi.

Freud, S. (2016d). Rüyaların Yorumu (S. Budak, Trans.). İstanbul: Öteki Yayınevi.

Freud, S. (2017a). Bir Yanılsamanın Geleceği (K. Şipal, Trans.). İstanbul: Say Yayınları.

Freud, S. (2017b). Mutluluk Dediğimiz Şey (P. Demirel, Trans.). İstanbul: Aylak Adam Yayınları.

Freud, S. (2017c). Totem ve Tabu (K. Şipal, Trans.). İstanbul: Say Yayınları.

Fromm, E. (1994). Sevginin ve Şiddetin Kaynağı (Y. Salman & N. İçten, Trans.). İstanbul: Payel Yayınevi.

Fromm, E. (2001). İtaatsizlik Üzerine (A. Sayın, Trans.). İstanbul: Kariyer Yayınları.

Fromm, E. (2003). Rüyalar Masallar Mitoslar (A. Arıtan & K. H. Ökten, Trans.). İstanbul: Arıtan Yayınevi.

Fromm, E. (2004a). Anaerkil Toplum ve Kadın Hakları (A. Doğangün, Trans.). İstanbul: Arıtan Yayınevi.

Fromm, E. (2004b). Freud Düşüncesinin Büyüklüğü ve Sınırları (A. Arıtan, Trans.). İstanbul: Arıtan Yayınevi.

Fromm, E. (2005). Psikanalizin Bunalımı (K. E. Kına, Trans.). İstanbul: Say Yayınları.

Fromm, E. (2006). Psikanaliz ve Din (E. Erten, Trans.). İstanbul: Say Yayınları.

Fromm, E. (2007). Sevme Sanatı (Ö. Saatçi-Karadana, Trans.). İzmir: İlya Yayıncılık.

Fuchs, C. (2014). Sosyal Medya: Eleştirel Bir Giriş (İ. Kalaycı & D. Saraçoğlu, Trans.). Ankara: NotaBene Yayınları.

Girgin, A. & Erkal, A. (2018). Düşünme ve Değerlendirme İpuçları. İstanbul: Salon Yayınları.

İnam, A. (2014). Teknoloji Benim Neyim Oluyor? Ankara: ODTÜ Yayıncılık.

Jung, C. G. (2016a). Kişiliğin Gelişimi (D. Olgaç, Trans.). İstanbul: Pinhan Yayıncılık.

Jung, C. G. (2016b). Analitik Psikoloji Üzerine İki Deneme (İ. H. Yılmaz, Trans.). İstanbul: Pinhan Yayıncılık.

Jung, C. G. (2016c). Analitik Psikoloji Sözlüğü (N. Nirven, Trans.). İstanbul: Pinhan Yayıncılık.

Köse, H. (2008). Lefebvre ve Modern Dünyada Gündelik Hayat. Gazi Üniversitesi İletişim Fakültesi Kuram ve Araştırma Dergisi. Güz, 27(2008), Ankara. 7–25.

McLuhan, M. & Fiore, Q. (2005). Yaradanımız Medya (Ü. Oskay, Trans.). İstanbul: Merkez Kitapçılık.

Oskay, Ü. (1994). Çağdaş Fantazya. Bilim-Kurgu ve Korku Sineması. İstanbul: Der Yayınları.

Övür, A. (2009). Facebook ve Simülasyon Evreni (Master's Thesis). Marmara Üniversitesi, Sosyal Bilimler Enstitüsü, İstanbul, Turkey.

Sanal Gerçeklik (VR) Nedir? (n.d.). Retrieved from https://www.istanbulbilisim.com/?act=ShowSSS&soru_ID=854 on 6 May 2018.

Semmelhack, P. (2013). Social Machines: How to Develop Connected Products That Change Customers' Lives. Hoboken, New Jersey: John Wiley & Sons.

Söğüt, F. (2015). Sanal Ortamda Aşkın Meta Olarak Pazarlanması; Online Arkadaşlık Siteleri Üzerine Bir İnceleme. In R. Çelik & S. Dalgalıdere (Eds.), Yeni ve Geleneksel Medya Okumaları (pp. 143–166). İstanbul: İskenderiye Kitap.

Yaylagül, L. (2006). Kitle İletişim Kuramları Egemen ve Eleştirel Yaklaşımlar. Ankara: Dipnot Yayınları.

Yengin, D. & Bayrak, T. (2017). Sanal Gerçeklik VR. İstanbul: Der Yayınları.

Yengin, D. ve Bayrak, T. (2018). Yeni Medya ve Sanal Gerçeklik. İstanbul: İstanbul Aydın Üniversitesi Yayınları.

Yengin, H. (1997). Bir İletişimsizlik Biçimi: Şiddet. İstanbul Üniversitesi İletişim Fakültesi Dergisi, 4, 147–218.

Yılmaz, H. R. (2010). Avatar: Fantazya Değil Mimesis. İletişim Çalışmaları Dergisi, 11, 154–174.

Deniz Yengin and Berkan Bayındır

Digitally Connected and/or Addicted

Abstract: This study questions the difference between being connected and addicted in a world where over half of the world with the population of 7.6 billion use the internet; more than half of 5 billion mobile users access the internet via their smart phones; last but not least nearly 360 thousand tweets are tweeted in a minute. Addiction is generally associated with uses and gratifications theory in communication studies. Media use gives individuals a chance to escape from the anxiety in the society they live in. The internet as a way of escaping from loneliness has reached a process during which it is firstly turned into a dependency, and gradually, into an addiction. The situation has now reached to such a serious level that rehabilitation centers have been established in a number of countries. It can be clearly seen that human-made technology has turned humans into mechanical slaves who need treatment. The study first gives a summary of the literature on dependency and addiction, then assesses the results of several studies conducted on the signs of addiction, and finally, enhances the terms "nomophobia" and "netlessphobia", which is the fear of lack of mobile phones and of the internet, respectively.

Keywords: technology addiction, digital addiction, internet addiction, leisure time, new media

Introduction

New media, social media, and the use of internet have now turned into a social habit. The use of social media, which stands out with several features, such as participation, openness, mutual conversation, community, and connectivity, is rapidly increasing day by day. The delicate line between being connected to social media and being addicted to it has exceeded. Addiction is often associated with the theory of uses and gratifications theory in communication studies. Mobile phones and social media which are used with these tools provide an opportunity to individuals for an escape. Addiction is an inevitable desire for an object, a person, or an entity and is the condition of being under the guidance of someone or something's volition (Uzbay, 2009). Experts state that new forms of addiction have emerged with the development of technology, and social media addiction is one of them.

After the emergence of the internet, the phenomenon of media addiction is being updated with the use of multi-channel communication platforms. Internet addiction disorder was named as internet addiction in 1995 by Ivan

Goldberg, who derived it from the notion of substance addiction in *Diagnostic and Statistical Manual of Mental Disorders*. Internet addiction is classified as a behavioral addiction. Extremism is the most decisive indicator in the classification of internet addiction. At this point, internet addiction means that people cannot control themselves while surfing the internet, and as a result, they experience some problems in their psychological, social, and academic lives. The social media usage frequency of individuals is increasing, the efforts to reduce this frequency are inconclusive and individuals feel deprivation when they cut off using it.

Being digitally connected means an individual is using the technology according to his/her own daily needs. As the interaction increases, technological developments are confronted as a deceptive fantasy and completely dazzle our eyes. Daily activities and requirements necessitate using the world which is converted into the digital. As a result, the individual uses the digital technology and is classified as "*digital connected*". However, the condition of being a digital addict is a behavioral technological addiction which is instigated by the feeling of incompleteness. The addicted generation consists of individuals who do not have social lives apart from the internet, who feel alone, altered or asocial when they are away from mobile devices, who follow closely all sorts of applications formed or developed in mobile phones, and want to be informed about all sorts of mobile innovations, who communicate with their friends through social media, and who form a new identity for themselves in social media.

The disorders called Nomophobia and Netlessphobia have reached worrying proportions. Nomophobia is the concern of being away from a mobile phone, which has emerged as a result of the development of smartphones and their integration with internet. Netlessphobia is the fear of being not able to reach the internet. These two disorders cause traumatic reactions that may result in mental breakdown. Technology produced by human has turned individuals into mechanical slaves and made them medically needy.

In this study, the technology-media-human interaction is questioned with its past and present. What has digital technology transformed the leisure time phenomenon into, and who controls the digital leisure time? The study is aimed to find the answers to these questions and examines how the approval stage in Everett's theory of "The Diffusion of Innovations", which consists of knowledge, persuasion, decision, acceptance and approval, has evolved into "The Process of Technology Addiction", by sub-classification of approval stage into "connected, addicted, and monotype". The study explains the difference between connected and addicted and assesses the results of several studies conducted towards symptoms of addiction.

Media-Technology-Human Interaction

Communication is regarded as one of the basic needs of humans. From past to the present day, the message transfer system has renewed itself, and the communication process is being socialized as a result of designing the medium with developing technologies. Source, object, environment and message are always being updated. But, depending on what? The answer is technology. Technique is the extension of humans' struggles against nature. The notion of technique as knowledge of achieving and producing something expresses a medium. However, the notion of technology derived from technique represents the social meaning and/or the socialization of that produced knowledge. In short, technology indicates the socialized knowledge. According to Ellul, technique resembles nothing but itself. It changes all the surroundings it interacts with, yet it is untouchable. Technique respects or worships no one and nothing; on the contrary, enslaves everyone and everything it interacts with. Moreover, the only thing that matters for technique is the product and production (Ellul, 2003: 342). Although the human really participates in the economy, technique causes him/her to participate in it not as human beings, but as things. Technique revolutionizes the production totally. Technique, which is designed and created by humans, makes a techno-copy of human life by transforming the technology. Humans as individuals, who cannot abandon current consumption behaviors, are strict followers of the products that technique has the monopoly on. Furthermore, humans are unsatisfied with this and send the technical content they gained to others who are at the same semantic code level. People who enjoy the functionality of the goods, and find them useful, get involved in a techno-social life as communities.

The new media technologies today exemplify that the one and only thing that matters for technique is the product and production. The reason of this is being under the pressure of technique people do not find conventional media enough and with the help of internet, they develop new media technologies in a very short period. Individuals, getting involved in each aspect of communication thanks to these technologies, suppress the fear of technology's pressure with continuous information flow provided by digital media. They become globalized as a result of the socialization of the produced knowledge and technically digitalized as techno-social individuals. The relationship between individual and technique always keeps up to date with production development assisted by technology, and now digitalized individual is emancipated whereas the mono-type consumption is discarded. Thus, technique directs people with the help of new media technologies and makes them consume current products. Individual, who has become the subject of techno-social life through technique, encounters

Tab. 1: Table of Communication Revolutions (Baldini, 2000)

Revolution	Medium	Period	Feature
Oral	Spoken Language	The emergence of human beings	The Power of Cognition
Chirographic	Written Language	B.C. 4th century	Manuscripts
Typographic	Printing press	15th century	The reproduction of books
Media	Telegram-Radio-Television	19th century	Mass communication

mechanical slavery. In mechanical slavery, people become cogs of the technical production and take a complementary position in the system by being integrated into technique (Lazzarato, 2016: 25). In this context, machine has been produced by people in line with the functionality of technique to provide the need of consumption. However, machine also shapes humans who produce it in accordance with its reasons of existence and directs the humans' consumption habits. This functionality of technique, on the one hand, reinforces the relationship between human and machine; on the other hand, by discarding the non-functional goods, makes people demand the current knowledge. Hence, the techno-social life is constantly shaped with information and the clusters of bit (binary digit) that represents the bottom units of information are specifically chosen for the technique in the name of this life. As the technique emerges, individuals gain the status of consumers in return for a fee and become members of that techno-social life. The techno-social life as a reflection of the social life metamorphoses with individuals' virtual identities in the new media technologies. Thanks to the anonymity which digital media serves, people can get involved in the consumption lines which they normally cannot get involved in the real social life and spread their knowledge without being censored in any kinds. In this context, individuals with their new virtual identities have discovered the liberal aspect of the techno-social life, developed new knowledge masses, and helped technique increase its effects on humans.

From this table, as Baldini states, it is understood that the technology determines the communication revolutions. Spoken language, written language, printing press, and telegram-radio-television, all makes the distinctions between revolutions. The way of human communication emerges according to medium which individuals use with the ongoing developments from the starting point of human life. The history of humanity starts with the invention of written language, and with this medium, information has become "collectable, transmittable, and storable". With the invention of printing press, the "diffusion" of stored information has been possible. The "processing" of information has been materialized as a result of the invention of computers. As it can be understood from Baldini's study, the development of communication media updates the communication processes of individuals. Walter Ong, Harold Innis, and Marshall McLuhan, who have studied about those mentioned approaches, ought to be assessed. The studies based on technology in communication are important research fields. The notion of technological determinism was first used by American sociologist and economist Thorstein Veblen.

Walter Ong dwells upon the relationship between spoken language and written language. Especially in this electronic era, it is seen that the difference between oral and written cultures has become even more significant. Ong, who describes the electronic era as "the era of second oral culture", stresses that existence is the era of the oral culture special to telephone, radio, and television which are based on the printing press technologies (1995: 15–25). Although oral narration can exist without written language, written narration cannot exist without oral narration. Words are based on oral communication; in contrary written language firmly restrains words to visual dimension. According to Ong, written language is a sort of technology, and it is artificial in all respects. Written language, as a sign of technological development, alters the medium of the message conveyed orally. Even though written language is not regarded as technology today, it had managed to be an important medium when it first existed with the use of alphabet. The printing press and computers can easily be qualified as technology. The most significant aspect of written language as a technology arises from its artificial nature. Contrary to the daily oral language, written language is totally artificial. In short, Ong highlights that reliability of space phenomenon has disappeared after the forms of written communication have become a part of oral communication. Ong, who has a critical approach to the written communication, states that storage of information will become easier with the written practices, yet the distances should not be so far during the communication process. The relationship between oral culture and time is very different from ours. During the periods when writing had not been invented yet, the concept of time was always present time and there was no past or future; also this approach sheds light on the concept of history in oral culture (Yengin, 2017: 28–32). Papyrus, parchment, and paper, the technological tools of written culture, have played a significant role on the transfer of information from past to present. Innis, who has studied on those technological tools, points out that the most important reason why communication network has developed is that written language has become widespread via printing press and electrical sources. The process of knowledge transfer, starting from manuscripts, has taken a shape through visual codes with the development of alphabet, and brought up a uniform, repeatable, and reproducible cultural reality. Innis clarifies how the new technology "competes with" the conventional information monopolies and how it emerges a new information monopoly ruled by another group. Innis tried to explain that communication technologies affect and shape societies' structures (Postman, 2004: 18). Innis thinks that oral tradition has a natural and incontestable competence (Innis, 2006: 95). Innis, who focuses on communication media, stresses that the transfer of message to generations has become easier with written language. The demand for parchment had increased because papyrus could not renew itself. Especially after paper has emerged, the transfer of information has become more widespread (Innis, 2006: 204). Paper as a medium enables people to convey a thought more cheaply and with a more economical material. According to Innis, papyrus, as a medium for written language, was very light compared to clay tablets. As a result of transferring the written language onto papyrus, the mobilization of thoughts had been enabled with the lightened medium. The thought became lighter; voice and thought took a form. According to Innis, who regards the alphabet as a technology, the monopolies had been sabotaged with the alphabet based on complex writing systems. The flexibility of the alphabet and its applicability to mechanization ease the convergence of printed words with oral tradition. Innis states that communication technology has created and changed the history of civilization. Even though communication technology is liberal by definition, it runs with a censored structure. Innis stresses that empires emerge with communication technologies, and the ones controlling those technologies can also dominate the world adding that communication mediums and technology are exactly inseparable. Developing and changing communication technology is the sign for ongoing reigns. The only changeable factor here is the identities of empires.

McLuhan's "Technological Determinism" approach emerges with renewal of the technology, and in this context the technology determines the masses. Technology means precision, and this precision is expressing one thing, one sense, one mental, or psychical process at a time. Once technology has enriched one of our senses, a new cultural transfer will arise along with the internalization of that new technology. McLuhan asserts that electrical technology has not substituted for an organ, but for the central nervous system itself; providing information as the primary product (Barbier & Lavenir, 2001: 303). According to him, the world is surrounded by images and messages, and one can immediately hear about the news all around the world, thanks to television (Yaylagül, 2010: 69). He states that technology, in a setting based on materiality, makes people feel defeated and left aside

Tab. 2: Table of Periodical Media Society by McLuhan (Laughey, 2007: 35)

Era	Forms of medium	Medium	Period
Tribe	Oral	Spoken Language	Before B.C. 1500s
End of Tribalization	Mechanic	Printing	1500–1900
Retribalization	Electrical	Television	After 1900s

their personality, and pushes them towards standardized lives, and in the end, directs them to fantasies. *Most technological tools are meant to develop the physical abilities of people; communication technology is an extension of thought, cognition and precious conceptual abilities of people. Hence, communication tools containing symbolic representation forms are actually the extensions of thought/brain* (Alemdar & Erdoğan, 1998: 146). According to McLuhan, since the various sub-systems of the social system interact with one another and all sub-systems require two-way flow of information in the electrical technology era, it is both possible and necessary to solve many problems in today's societies. McLuhan concludes that technology is beneficial and necessary for the social system, so it is possible to be optimistic based on technological determinism.

The forms of media used in the change of eras are noteworthy. Different mediums were seen in each era. Spoken language, printing, and television directed the periodical changes and developments. As Innis also states, the tools of the empire effect and direct our lives (Yengin: 2015: 58). McLuhan argues that the medium is important, not the content of the message and he supports this assumption with technology. He stresses that the technological structure is decisive, and technology has considerable power that can create new societies and life conditions (Yengin, 2017: 28–32).

Humans' struggles with nature and their environments create new dynamics. These dynamics have become inseparable parts of people with time. The phenomena of technique and technology are signs of those dynamics. All information created by trial and error to fulfill the needs is addressed as technique, and the extension of it is defined as technology. As Atabek also notes, technique is "the knowledge of achieving something" whereas technology is "the socialization and gaining a social value of that produced and/or achieved knowledge". Techniques get permanent statuses psychically in communicational issues. In this survival struggle, the notion of technique has successfully become the fixture of individuals at first, and respectively, society and global structure afterwards. Technique that exists through the cultures of the societies is an inseparable part of today's lifestyle. Technology is transferred through culture, expressed, and used through production. Technique has formed a dynamic and permanent structure with the relationship between technique and economy. Technology reveals the way of human beings' struggle with nature and the production process they pursue in their lives, thus reveals the formation of social relations and the style of mental designs emerge from those relations (Mosco & Fuchs, 2014: 152). At this point, to define the economy and economy-politics in a right way and assess the system of capitalism has become important. Capitalism considers the economy in the center as a system of capital production, where the means of production are owned and controlled by private property, economic activities are carried out in order to gain profits and capital is owned by capital owners (Odyakmaz & Acar, 2008: 71). In this context, the economy is subjected to regulations aimed at maintaining and improving the functioning of capitalism. The capitalist economic order engaged with technique designs the technology to shape the consumption society and guide the society's demands. In this case, technically equipped people are in an effort to maintain the economy politics in favor of the present order by producing machines, and also to reduce the time of production. As a result, people who implement technology through mechanical slavery in all aspects of their lives preserve the flow of capitalist capital for the continuation of this slavery tradition. *"Mechanical slavery takes the place of "human slavery" regimes of the old imperial systems (Egypt, China, etc.) and therefore it is a mode of command, regulation and governance supported by technology, in this way it represents one of the authenticities of capitalism"* (Lazzarato, 2016: 25). People who have shaped their lifestyles with mechanical slavery use mass media and new media technologies when they want to get up-to-date technique. However, information sources have always been monopolized throughout history. Formatting, and especially designed information, guides the individual users and determines the developmental course of the technology. Nevertheless, the informational monopolies are eventually condemned to be destructed. Because apart from being the recipient of knowledge, people want to be involved in the formation of knowledge.

The world that people have built with their own hands contains much more variety of products than the necessary to meet basic human needs. This diversity can be described as a result of technological evolution, since the continuity of things produced by people keeps its existence; innovation becomes an essential part of the world that people have built up, and the process of selection is functioning to choose between new products to multiply and add new things to the store of products (Basalla, 2013: 47). In the context of these explained technology

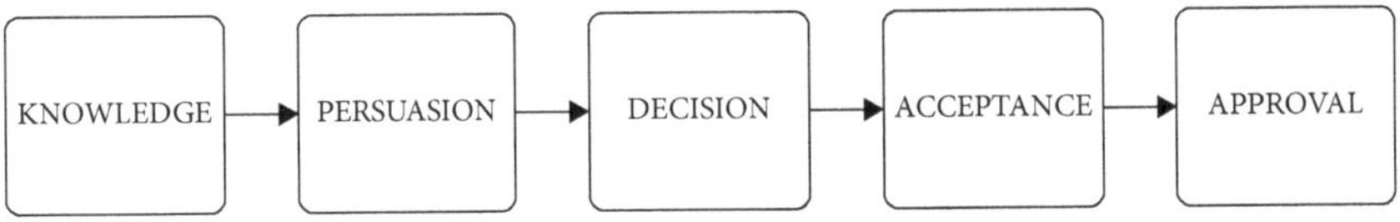

Fig. 1: Diffusion of Innovations (Innovation-Decision Process) (Rogers, 1995: 165).

definitions and approaches, it is necessary to focus on how technology, which determines and transforms society, is used and diffused by masses.

In the literature "*The Diffusion Theory of Innovations*" is defined as the concept of new product, new market, new advertising and distribution, etc. systems, as "innovation". The theory was popularized by Rogers Everett in the 1960s, and in 1962 it was published in the name of "*Diffusion of Innovations*". Rogers refers to the theory of diffusion of innovations as changes in the individual or social system following the adoption or rejection of an innovation. *These are knowledge, persuasion, decision, acceptance and approval.* Rogers considers the individuals' acceptance stages of innovation in five categories:

Knowledge is the first stage and the individual encounters the innovation but has no knowledge on that. Furthermore, s/he is not aware of the innovation. At the stage of persuasion, the individual who is actively involved in innovation is not looking for information and detail. During decision stage, the individual uses the innovation to inquire about its advantages and disadvantages, and as a result, accepts or rejects it. The individual might make a decision about the usefulness of the innovation and engage in a deeper research about the innovation. At the final stage, approval, the individual has made a final decision on the product. The results of researches which are conducted with Rogers' model demonstrate that mass media plays an important role in the diffusion and acceptance of innovations in society, but there it has no strong influence on the approval stage. In this process, the individual's effect shows great interoperability (Rogers, 1995: 165–205). In conclusion, technology is being decisive and directive at every stage of our life. As being the most popular medium of today, new media also represents technology. By defining the new media in this context, it is possible to observe the diversity that this tool has added to the communication process.

New Media as Technology

The need is the core of the invention. Our needs and necessities direct the technology. Entities have managed to become the most important tools of human beings in life during the struggle against nature (Basalla, 2013: 18). As the technical level of these tools increases, each object evolves into a new tool. The technological invention always leads to a distinctive progression in the evolving product. Developments in the field of technology directly contribute to the improvement of our material, social, cultural, and spiritual life; thus speeds up the growth of civilization. Progress gained in the field of technology, and accordingly in civilization, can be measured precisely with speed, efficiency, power, and the other quantitative measures. The origin, direction, and effect of technological change are completely under human control (Basalla, 2013: 324).

Science focuses on knowledge for exploration, while technology focuses on necessary knowledge development. Technological innovations put leverage on the system and thus, necessitate transformation. According to Postman, as technology develops, both the winners and losers of the system changes. From the combination of the online world with the offline physical world, social reflections emerge. Socialization is realized with the internet, which is an unlimited technology-based global network. According to Chayko, internet, mobile communication, and social media network are the carriers of the global revolution (Chayko, 2018: 40). As Gibson points out, the digital experiences of individuals, behind the scenes of all computer screens, are real and precise. Any form, texture, shape, depth, and details that the individuals actually use are revised while transferring them into the digital.

According to McLuhan, the right lobe of the human brain operates in verbal whereas the left lobe operates in visual format. He considers that technological development is shaped by this separation. In this context, McLuhan indicates that the auditory space and the visual space cannot be separated from one another, and thus the technology has also developed sticking to this separation, that is the reason why human is whole with technology. According to McLuhan, the visual space used by technology is a side effect of the monotonous, persistent and fragmented character of the phonetics. Additionally, technologies are metaphors just like words. Similarly, they transform users until new relationships are established between the user and his/her environment (McLuhan, 2001: 33). In this sense, as the left lobe of human beings' brain supports visual format, it is seen that the virtual reality embraced by technology today is shaped with this format. However, McLuhan indicates that people, who mostly use their left lobe, will show aggression as main mental qualification. Accordingly, the technique which is a human product will be in an aggressive attitude. The technology resulting from that technique, therefore, will also have aggressive motives. McLuhan states that there are four senses in the nature (sight, hearing, touch and taste). All technology is an extension of these four talents. The technique's existence is based on these four senses, and it plays an important role in people's technology management. In this context, technologies will occupy the inner peace of people by filling every moment when they are awake and there will be moments when people need somewhere to hide (McLuhan, 2001: 232). Since all the services provided by technology in the electronic era can be accessed everywhere, centralization becomes impossible; humans develop technology in the sake of collecting information from everywhere. However, what matters is not the content and the quality of the content provided by the technology, but the technology itself. This is because the technology is at the stage of guiding human life, and it is important to understand what the message sent by that technology is. Technology as a message all alone takes place in human life; according to this, technology is a scale, a step, or a change of the attitude that is embedded in human relations and continues developing as an extension of an individual's four senses.

The most important message presented by a technological tool is how it affects human life. Because technology is not innocent, and it will definitely make people dependent on itself. McLuhan explains how media technology, which is the main technological development, shapes society, with the assumption that the medium is the message. According to him, people have developed the technologies by imitating the facts of the previous time. This technology is analyzed through the message it gives, so that the developed technology can be explained, and the codes of the messages that are emitted by it can be predicted beforehand. McLuhan states that communication tools, which are the product of technology and developed by people to reduce the communication process, should be classified so that the content of the messages given by the tools can easily be understood. Accordingly, technological tools are separated from each other as cold and hot tools. Tools that appeal to only one sense of the individual are described as hot (film, photography, radio, etc.), and those that appeal to multiple senses are described as cold tools (television, telephone, comic books, etc.). In this context, technology serves as an extension of humans addressing to their senses and this structure is dominant. As McLuhan examines the place of technology in humans' life which is determined by the technique, he also explains at what degree humans need technology, adding that this process has reached to an irreversible point. The new media has managed to get involved in humans' lives with its features like being user-based, digital, interactive, hypertext, virtual and networked. These features show us the distinction between the conventional and new. Especially digital coding is an important feature in qualifying the media as "new". In a short time period, a second space emerges by coding the data which has started with bits.

According to Van Dijk, by using "*integrated, interactive and digital coding*", the transition from the 20th century to the 21st was provided. In this respect,

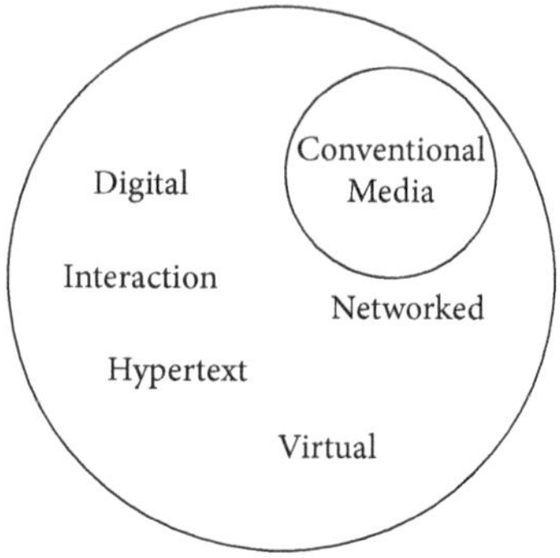

Fig. 2: New Media Features (Yengin, 2015: 140).

it is easy to make a distinction between the old and new (2006: 9). In simple terms, the new media set also contains the traditional. In this work, traditional and new forms of media are complementary to each other. Features like being digital, interactive, hyper-texted, networked, and virtual have enabled the media to be new, and they are placed in that set. At this point, the most important point is the position of the traditional media within the set. Traditional media takes place in the new media set. Within this set, only the other new media features are separated from each other. The new notion continues its way by including the traditional. With the internet, time and space could have been restructured. Technology's aim is to process the information systematically. Along with the digital technology, instead of complexity, interfaces that can deal with much work with little information are created. In today's informatics era, it is important to reach information and control it. Knowledge is easy to reach for users, but it is not easy for them to update and share information. The new media, which works as "*Hold-drag-and-drop*", makes it possible for the user to interfere with the content. In order to explain the transformation of conventional media as new media, the concept of digitalization needs to be completely understood. With the internet, time and space could have been restructured. Technology's aim is the systematically process of information. Along with the digital technology, interfaces that can deal with much work with little information are created. Without data it is not possible to produce content. With the developing technology, the data has become even more valuable. While we are producing data, consuming, managing, and making money; we are unaware that we become a monotype and enslaved over time, as Marcuse states. In the diffusion of innovations theory, the integration into life practices in new media provides

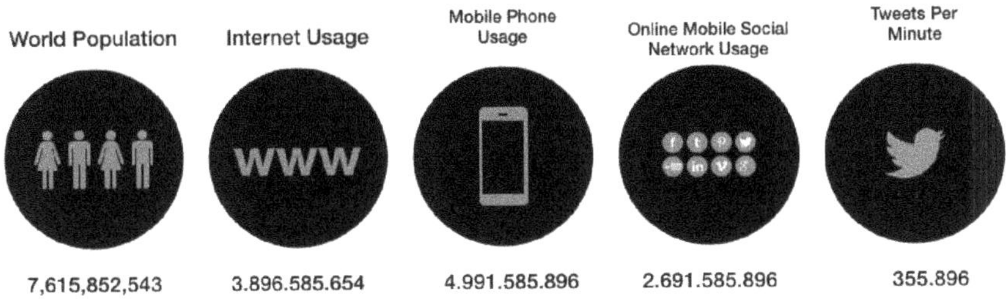

Fig. 3: Data on General Internet Usage (Worldometers, n.d.).

the time and space convenience after knowledge, persuasion, decision, acceptance, and approval stages. The cases of being connected, addicted, and monotype can now be explained with the digitization process.

Digitally Connected or/and Digitally Addicted

In the world, more than half of the 7.6 billion people use the internet. Approximately 5 billion people have mobile phones, and more than 2.5 billion have access to internet via mobile phones. Therefore, one-third of the world's population is mobile internet users. We can easily observe that the digital transformation happens rapidly, from the continuous use of the digital communication process. Within a minute, about 360 thousand tweets are shared. Daily data exchange now takes place with digital communication. At this point, *in 2012, the International Society for Technology in Education has also included the concept of digital citizenship among the qualifications for school administrators, teachers and students. According to the definition of the International Technology Education Society, the "digital citizenship" standards of students are as follows: Students understand humanitarian, cultural and social issues related to technology and act accordingly in legal and ethical terms. In this respect, they advocate and enforce the safe, legal and responsible use of information and technology. They demonstrate a positive attitude towards the use of technology to collaborate, learn and promote productivity, and demonstrate personal responsibility for lifelong learning and leadership for digital citizenship*. In the context of digitally established communication, each transaction is recorded as digital data. This means that individuals leave their digital footprints for every transaction they make.

Social media has become a social habit. The social media is used according to the needs and interests of the individuals, and every citizen is involved in it. The technique, which played a major role in transforming technology from tool to aim after the Industrial Revolution, has carried out this function under human control. However, human production technology, as always, brings along the problems of addiction. The features of participation, openness, conversation, community, and connectivity increase usage of the social media. At this point, addiction is often associated with the uses and gratification theory in communication studies. Individual's escape from unease of the society materializes through the use of the media. Therefore, mobile phones as a new media and social media used with these tools are the most important ways of getting away from the struggles in the society.

Addiction is the inevitable desire for an object, person, and entity or else being guided by another will (Uzbay, 2009). Uzbay also states that addiction is a certain problematic situation or a desire that cannot be prevented, although it is harmful to people's mental, physical health and social life. Only three of the following symptoms are sufficient to put the diagnosis of dependency. These are; *increase in the duration of use, feeling deprivation when a shortage happens in the usage, continual efforts to reduce the duration of use, decrease in social activities because of the usage, and continual usage despite the physical problems*. Three main situations come up when the abovementioned cases are evaluated in terms of addiction. These are *the inevitable desire for usage, the increase in the duration of use and the lack of physical and psychological requirements*. Addiction can be classified as cognitive, emotional, and behavioral. The first one is the addiction to information; the second one is the addiction to socialization and escape; and the last one is the addiction to instrumental and operational situations. Ball-Rokeach states five important qualities of the individuals' media addiction: structural (being connected to political, economic, cultural and the other systems), content (the nature of social environment), media (sharing and quality of messages), interpersonal environment (personal relationship network), and individual factors (individual's target). In the context of these qualities, Ball-Rokeach explains that the high degree of addiction to media eases to change the individuals' feelings and thoughts (Severin & Tankard, 1994: 460–464). Typology of addiction relations obtained as a result of individual and social evaluations of understanding, orientation and play processes is used to explain the communication process that individuals develop with the media. It is highly important for individuals to understand, perceive, and describe the environment in their struggle with the nature. Individuals rely on the resources of the media system to materialize their personal goals, such as understanding who they are, how they grow, and change. While doing this, social interaction and individual actions become decisive. Individual orientation is defined as action orientation,

Tab. 3: Typology of Addiction Relations (DeFleur and Ball-Rokeach, 1989)

INDIVIDUAL	SOCIAL
UNDERSTANDING	
Personal development and self-understanding	Information about the world, society and about interpreting them
ORIENTATION (TENDENCY)	
To decide what to buy, how to wear and how to keep thin	To get tips on how to behave when new and difficult situations are encountered
PLAY	
To relax when you are alone or decide what to do	To go to a cinema or listen to music with family or friends

and social orientation is defined as interaction orientation. Individuals who refer to information resources of the media system can interact with others for social orientation. In order to escape from social and daily problems, individuals may tend to entertainment or play. The aesthetics, entertainment, and relaxation functions of the media encourage the individual to use these systems. It is an important feature of this game to share comments about a series that individuals have watched as someone having information about it in order to increase their social interaction. Each game played at this point represents culture.

Addiction is often used to refer to physical attachment to an item. The media dependency phenomenon is updated with the use of multi-channel communication platforms with the emergence of the internet. Social media and the internet have brought many new innovations together that rescue people from being local and make them global. While the individuals have difficulty in accessing the people whom they are interested, with the social media, they have a chance to engage with interest-oriented groups of friends. Experts state that with the development of technology, new addiction types have emerged nowadays, and social media addiction is one of them. It is stated that among this addiction type with the highest risk of being seen between 12 and 18 age group, males show 2–3 times more addictive behaviors than females.

The Internet addiction disorder was named by Ivan Goldberg in 1995 as an addiction to the internet, derived from the substance abuse of the Diagnostic and Statistical Manual of Mental Disorders. Internet addiction as a behavioral dependency includes the elements of clarity, moody, tolerance, withdrawal symptoms, contradictions, and relapses. As a result of making communication practices via the internet, addiction is triggered. Most researchers, such as Griffiths (1998) and Young (1998), state that problems arise related with business, family, school, and friends because of internet addiction. Extremism is the most important determinant in the classification of internet addiction. At this point, internet addiction means that one cannot control himself/herself on internet usage and as a result, s/he experiences problems in his/her psychological, social, and academic life. Being addicted to imaginary world of media has always existed. But when we compare the addiction to new and old media, it is understood that new media makes people to be connected itself in longer periods and it has the feature which draws people into itself more. A television addict can go back to the reality at least during the commercials and needs to wait a week for the new episode whereas one who watches the series on the internet can possibly watch the whole season in one or two days without stopping. From this point of view, it is possible to say that old media's anesthetization period is limited, and its dose is light whereas new media's anesthetization dose and its potential of taking someone out of reality is higher (Övür, 2017: 34).

Internet-addicted digital migrants and digital locals in general would exhibit intense interest towards the internet, anxious posture in the non-internet environment, escape from responsibility, and exceeding the period of use. As a means of escaping from solitude, the internet is gradually moving toward a process of being connected and then addicted over the time. The most prominent features that have emerged in many surveys for addiction statements are *unable to put limit, keep using in spite of harm, anxiety in unusual times, and severe reactions.* At this point, the phenomenon of a disease means the state of disability and discomfort by the occurrence of some changes in the organism. In this regard, digital disease is the deterioration of health as a result of some changes in the organism because of using digital media.

It is possible to give some examples to the digital diseases. Discomforts targeting at the mental health of people called Nomophobia and Netlessphobia have reached threatening proportions. Nomophobia is the deprivation of a mobile phone, which has emerged as a result of the development of smartphones and the integration of smartphones with internet (Alter, 2018: 33). Netlessphobia is the fear of staying without the internet. These two disorders severely threaten an individual's health profile and cause traumatic reactions to mental decline in individuals. In this context, rehabilitation centers have been established in many countries. Aim of the centers is to protect and treat the individuals against the adverse effects of the internet and the mobile phones. When this situation is examined, it seems that the human-made technology has turned the human beings into mechanical slaves and made them need medical care now. Although the technique seems to be taking some precautions as a result of impaired mental health (such as night light application on Apple's current phones, etc.), the number of people complaining of disorders, such as Nomophobia and Netlessphobia, is increasing day by day. Wi-Fi addiction is to feel nervous in an environment where there is no access to internet. The most obvious indicator of addiction here is that one feels nervous. Besides addiction, the internet can also cause harmful effects such as heart rhythm disturbance, inability to focus, lack of attention, migraine, insomnia, Parkinson disease by sending electromagnetic waves to the individuals. If the nomophobia is reinforced by stress or panic in case of being away from smartphones, and if one cannot detect the events in the environment, s/he feels the need of continuously controlling the mobile device, this means that the patient is still in the first stage. As the use of smart mobile devices increases, they excrete the feeling of happiness in the brain. Well-known scientists have consolidated this fact with mobile devices and dopamine-releasing hormone. If the hormones that give the person a sense of happiness are released when the person's device receives a notification, this indicates that addiction phase is increasing. It should be mentioned that users must be aware of how much time they spend on smart mobile devices and control themselves for conscious use in order to get rid of Nomophobia or its symptoms that are confronted as a cerebral disorder. Nomophobia-aggrieved individuals are sleeping with their phones, check their phones for 15 minutes as soon as they wake up, and as a result, they spend a month in a year on a mobile phone.

It is necessary to ask the following questions to ourselves. If we are doing at least half of the actions mentioned in these questions, then we may have become addicted:

- *if you are mostly trying to handle your daily work from the internet,*
- *if you have given up your hobbies,*
- *if you are glued to your mobile phone,*
- *if you carry spare charges,*
- *if you look at your phone immediately after you wake up in the morning,*
- *if your fear of being without news has increased,*
- *if you have begun to neglect your duties and responsibilities related with your business and/or your home,*
- *if you are sleepless because of spending time on the social media,*
- *if you think you are apart from your friends.*

Taking these explanations into consideration, the "Technology Addiction Process" is being renewed by the additions to Everett's "Diffusion of Innovations" process. The socialization of the technique, which is the knowledge of getting something, is presented as technology. At this point, socialized knowledge needs to fulfill the processes of diffusion of innovations theory.

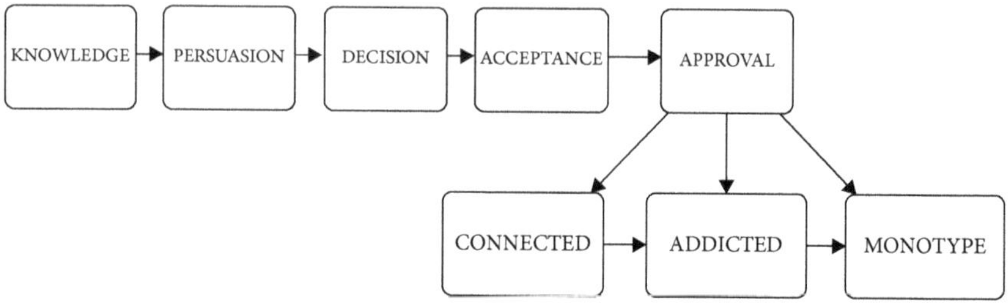

Fig. 4: Process of Technology Addiction (Adapted from Rogers, 1995: 165).

The subject has become so popular that even a mobile application related with this has been developed. Through this application which is called "Moment", people can observe their own usage. Moment application monitors all activities and watches the users except for listening to music and speaking on the phone. Two data are important here: the duration of phone usage and the number of contacts with the phone. At the approval level, the frequency of usage determines the situations of being connected, addicted, and monotype conditions. The procedure is performed by subtracting an average sleep time of 8 hours over 24 hours. The remaining 16 hours and within this time the usage period of technology is classified.

Contemporary mass consumption is a whole of spare applications; every consumer is an unpaid household worker who works to produce individuals as masses. Individuals consume leisure products at the highest level. The colonization of leisure time by television can be seen as another manifest of the historical process in which leisure time has been turned into a commodity and seized again by the powers in control of the necessity area. For the great majority of people, leisure time has turned into a time for television rather than a "time for higher activities" for the full development of the individual, as Marx points out (Şahin & Robinson, 1980: 94). The individual is amused and impersonated under the guise of entertainment and debarred from his/her human features. The individual is an apathetic and a passive consumer outside the world, not inside it. The individuals experience the world through images (Yengin, 2015: 211–257). As a result of reproduction of real events, the distinction between the reality and the image of reality is suppressed. The main purpose of the information, entertainment, and educational material on the media is to attract attention to the products and services that are advertised. People who pursue their personal interests and benefits in their leisure time do not get involved in any social and political activities. According to Smythe, the mass media was developed by monopoly capitalism.

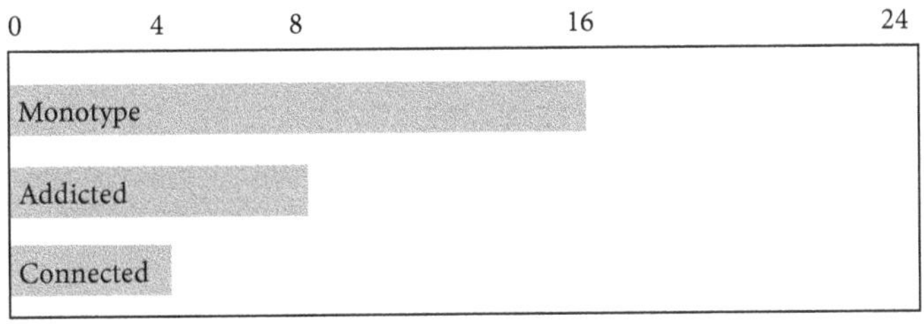

Fig. 5: Durations of Technology Use.

The aim is to teach people consumption, to support the system with votes and taxes, to build public opinion, and to make profits (Yaylagül, 2010: 164).

Technology has transformed people's access to leisure time and changed their experiences about leisure time. Computers, smartphones, and tablets, along with other technological devices, have become the perfect screen of the leisure environment (Blanco, 2014: 191–193). Briefly, digital leisure time means that an individual is doing his/her daily activities by using digital media. With its digital feature, the new media is constantly being used by the individuals and the individuals can live online. Physical identity and digital identity can work together. However, Bauman's liquid modernity theory keeps the individuals under control. Therefore, the individuals adopt their digital identities more. This ownership especially transforms the leisure activities of the individuals, and the habits are updated along with the transformation. The purpose of the mass broadcasting was to get the consumers' attention somehow and get them on the time train and keep them in that train as long as possible. As for new broadcasting systems, as well as digital platforms (or "online video streaming" platforms), and Netflix, for sure, the purpose is to catch the consumers with appealing invitations, and never let them go, if possible (Şahin, 2019).

At this point, in the approval step, "Technology Addiction Process" can be categorized according to the frequency of usage with statuses as; connected-addicted-monotype. As shown in Fig. 5, the use of digital technology for 0–4 hours is regarded as connected, 4–8 hours as addicted, and 8–16 hours as monotype. The fact that individuals are connected or addicted to technology is classified on the basis of the duration of technology usage.

As Debord (2006: 42) notes, the statement "show is the watchman of sleep" most obviously demonstrates the situation that we are currently living in. The show makes sense of visible events by combining the differences between them. Technology-based new media both controls and directs us. Postman, like Debord, defends the view that the visuals used with communication tools make everything ordinary. At this point, it becomes almost compulsory for the consumer to perform consumption and production in the digital environment during that show bombardment. Therefore, everyday activities and requirements necessitate using the world transmitted into the digital. Hence, the individuals use digital technology and are classified as "digitally connected".

Being digital addict, on the other hand, is a non-chemical but a behavioral technology addiction that emerges with a feeling of incompleteness. The addicted generation includes individuals who do not have a social life other than the Internet; who feels themselves alone, metamorphosed, or asocial when they are away from mobile devices; who follow closely all kinds of applications produced or being developed on the phone and who want to be informed about any mobile innovation; who communicate with their friends via social media; and who have formed a new identity in the social media. These people, who frequently log in and log out social media applications in daily life, keep these applications active, feel disconnected from the reality of everyday life while experiencing the virtual reality, and feel themselves excluded from the society, fill their missing side with mobile devices, and feel satisfied. These people, who are caught up in mobile devices, have become comfortable in expressing themselves in mobile environment without creating eye contact, even though they are shy in social life and there is no need for labor or responsibility. Through their mobile devices, they can also be whoever they want to be and give their selves the status they desire with new identities.

Conclusion

The face-to-face communication of the individual in society continues through social media. This is a simple indication of the integrated communication process in traditional and new media. However, the request for communication happens instantaneously and placeless in digital media, like in traditional one. At this point, the technology which individuals often use triggers addiction. Kevin Kelly emphasizes that everything that is impossible in theory become possible in practice when one connects to the internet (2010: 17). He means that there is only a single global machine and that everything is transferred to and shared with this machine. 100 billion clicks are done per day, and there are 55 trillion connections between networks. In addition, this machine uses 5 % of the global system's electricity. By the time 2040, the total processing capacity of the machine will have exceeded the processing capacity of the whole humanity. Clay Shirky, a techno optimist, predicts that more information will spontaneously turn into more collective action. According to the optimists, democracy will come along spontaneously with the social media. In contrary, techno pessimist Evgeny Morozov states that social networks such as Facebook and Twitter are used for entertainment, but they are based on daily shares rather than political organizations, and that this technology enhances the possibilities of the state's security devices monitor the people. In his study titled Net Delusion, Morozov states that the new technology provides more control for the user over the communication process. The communication process that begins with spoken language has left the place to the digital systems today. The communication medium that are changing with technological developments as a result of the information age keeps maintaining as natural extensions of the traditional communication environment.

Technology directs and shapes the history. The hypothesis of Innis' "those who possess communication also rules the world" has become more evident in today's environment. In global culture formation, technology-based communication mediums facilitate the control of individuals by the system together with digital transformation. Because the individuals are coded with numbers and they represent themselves in the virtual media. At this point, it becomes almost compulsory to use new media. This logic of "there is no place for the ones who do not use and learn the new media" is imposed on the individuals. Requests that guide the information are formed through work, language, and power. Habermas, with that statement, advocates the argument that those who have knowledge also govern society. Technique and science are guided by the points of view desired by ideologies and produced towards this direction because science and technique have become the most important powers. In the developed countries, especially science and technology are steadily directed. New technologies are supported, produced, and managed by the global system in the light of new information. Technology culture directs people to believe via vision. This assumption becomes seriously dangerous if the information is prepared by certain people and is transmitted in an ideological way. Information is transformed into an ideological basis and presented to individuals in that way. This situation is used to direct and control individuals rather than informing them. Individuals gladly use this new media. People are voluntarily involved in all kinds of activities. The individuals working in this media copy what the others do. Imitation is becoming widespread, and the things are becoming ordinary, even though they seem to be special. The approach of one-dimensional society society that Herbert Marcuse (2010) emphasizes is fully materialized with the new media. What we believe is decided by the rulers of the new media and presented to the masses. Today's society works for pleasure and entertainment, and it is being directed to do so because the individuals are shaped not by their own decisions, but by the decisions of the global system. As a result of that shaping process, individuals are getting similar to one another. Digital media makes us transparent. In Foucault's approach, his study titled "Birth of the Prison", everyone in the prison is being controlled and monitored. However, the observer and the controller cannot certainly be seen by the individuals. Individuals are easily seen and watched in the virtual world they represent by their digital identities. The individuals are unaware of the situation in which they live and, in this context, they actually live in a fully transparent prison.

Over the years, humans, who aimed to reduce communication in a shorter period of time, first created the Conventional Media and then headed for New Media technologies with the help of the internet. The main purpose in all these developments is to ensure that the communication process is successfully completed. In this sense, it seems that everything consists of texts for the individuals. These texts are transferred to the target through the communication process. In these transmissions, the channel or medium has a significant position. Huizinga describes the game as "something unreal, but, at the same time, can badly and entirely pull the actors in the game from the beginning to the end, while both the freedom of working consciously continue outside and the ordinary life, as it is the current one continues" (Huizinga, 1995: 13). Jesper Juul, on the other hand, describes the game as "transferable activity that has variable and numerical results from rules, different consequences are assigned to different values, the player has endeavoured to influence the outcome, and the resultant emotionally focused outcome is the transferable activity" (2005: 36). The game is an activity that is done willingly and regularly at a certain time and place.

In this sense, game means unreal that has some rules and entries-exits within predetermined boundaries. With each technical development, the toys of the individual are being renewed and the individuals are being remodeled by using these toys. As a result, the life as a play, which is constantly played by individuals, has paved the way to the foundation for the emergence of technology. From this point of view, the development of the internet, in the context of the technological determinism approach, expresses the transition to the Semantic Web with the intelligent data (Yengin, 2017). With semantic data, which can think and personalize, we will not have to think about many things in the near future.

Bibliography

Alemdar, K. & Erdoğan, İ. (1998). Başlangıcından Günümüze İletişim Kuram ve Araştırmaları. Ankara: MY Yayınları.

Alter, A. (2018). Karşı Konulmaz (D. İrengün, Trans.). İstanbul: Paloma Yayınları.

Barbier, F. & Lavenir, C. (2001). Diderot'dan İnternete Medya Tarihi. İstanbul: Okyanus Yayın.

Baldini, M. (2000). İletişim Tarihi (G. Batuş, trans.). İstanbul: Avcıol.

Basalla, G. (2013). Teknolojinin Evrimi. Ankara: Doğu Batı Yayınları.

Bauman, Z. (1998). Globalization: The Human Consequences. Cambridge: Polity Press; Oxford: Blackwell Publishers Ltd.

Blanco, A. (2014). Dijital Çağda Boş Zamanın Dönüşümü, In B. Çoban (Ed.), Sosyal Medyada Devrim (pp. 185–199). İstanbul: Su Yayınları.

Chayko, M. (2018). Süperbağ(lantı)lı: İnternet, Dijital Medya & Tekno-Sosyal Hayat. İstanbul: Der Yayınları.

Debord, G. (2006). Gösteri Toplumu. İstanbul: Ayrıntı Yayınları.

DeFluer, M. L. & Ball-Rokeach, S. (1989). Theories of Mass Communication. New York: Pearson.

Ellul, J. (2003). Teknoloji Toplumu (M. Ceylan, trans.). İstanbul: Bakış Yayınları.

Fuchs, C. (2014). Social Media: A Critical Introduction. London: Sage.

Griffiths, M. D. (1998). Internet Addiction: Does it really exist? In Gackenbach (ed.), Psychology and the Internet: Intrapersonal, Interpersonal and Transpersonal Applications (pp. 61–75). New York: Academic Press.

Huizinga, J. (1995). Homo Ludens Oyunun Toplumsal İşlevi Üzerine Bir Deneme (M.A. Kılıçbay, Trans.). İstanbul: Ayrıntı Yayınları.

İnnis, H. (2006). İmparatorluk ve İletişim Araçları. Ankara: Ütopya Yayınevi.

Juul, J. (2005). Half-Real: Video Games Between Real Rules and Fictional Worlds. Massachusetts: The MIT Press.

Kelly, K. (2010). What Technology Wants. New York: Penguin Books.

Laughey, D. (2007). Key Themes in Media Theory. New York: Open University Press.

Lazzarato, M. (2016). Göstergeler ve Makineler (F.N. Demirci, Trans.). İstanbul: Otonom Yayıncılık.

Marcuse, H. (2010). Tek-Boyutlu İnsan: İleri İşleyim Toplumunun İdeolojisi Üzerine İncelemeler. İstanbul: İdea Yayınevi.

McLuhan, M. (2001). Global Köy. İstanbul: Scala Yayıncılık.

Mosco, V. & Fuchs, C. (2014). Marx Geri Döndü: Medya, Meta ve Sermaye Birikimi. Ankara: NotaBene Yayınları.

Odyakmaz, A. N. & Acar, N. O. (2008). İletişim Sözlüğü. İstanbul: Babil Yayınları.

Ong, W. (1995). Sözlü ve Yazılı Kültür. İstanbul: Metis Yayıncılık.

Övür, A. (2017). Diseases and the Possible Effects that the New Media Brought into the Digitalizing World. Communication and Technology Congress 2017, İstanbul, 22–23 Kasım 2017, İstanbul Aydın Üniversitesi, CTC Conference Proceedings Book, ISSN: 978-88-87729-44-3, (http://www.edlearning.it/ebook/AY11.pdf) (Conference Proceedings Citation Index- Social Science & Humanities) 20–36.

Postman, N. (2004). Yeni Dünya Düzeni: Teknopoli. İstanbul: Gelenek Yayıncılık.

Rogers, E. M. (1995). Diffusion of Innovations. New York: Free Press.

Severin, W. & Tankard, J. (1994). İletişim Kuramları: Kökenleri, Yöntemleri ve Kitle İletişim Araçlarında Kullanımları (A.A. Bir & S. Sever, trans.). Eskişehir: Anadolu Üniversitesi Yayınları.

Şahin (2019, March 4). Zaman ve Roman. Netizenlist. Retrieved from http://www.netizenlist.com/zaman-ve-roman/ on 10 January 2019.

Şahin, H. & Robinson, J.P. (1980). Beyond the Realm of Necessity: Television and The Colonization of Leisure. Media, Culture and Society, 3, 85–95.

Van Dijk, J. (2006). The Network Society: Social Aspects of New Media, 2nd ed. London: Sage Publications.

Worldometers. (n.d.). Retrieved from https://www.worldometers.info/ on 16 April 2018

Yaylagül, L. (2010). Kitle İletişim Kuramları: Egemen ve Eleştirel Yaklaşımlar. Ankara: Dipnot Yayınları.

Yengin, D. (2015). Yeni Medya ve Dokunmatik Toplum. İstanbul: Derin Yayınları.

Yengin, D. (2017). İletişim Çalışmalarında Araştırma Yöntemleri ve Uygulamaları. İstanbul: Der Yayınları.

Young, K. (1998). Internet Addiction: The Emergence of a New Clinical Disorder. Cyberpshchol Behavior, 1, 237–244.

Uzbay, T. (2009). Madde Bağımlılığının Tarihçesi, Tanımı, Genel bilgiler ve Bağımlılık Yapan Maddeler, Meslek İçi Sürekli Eğitim Dergisi, 21, 5–15.

Didem Ataman Yengin

Digital Game Addiction

Abstract: Digital game addiction creates a danger which is threatening our future, i.e., our children. Parents who cannot take their children to open air and lead them to play outside because of the insufficient playgrounds as a result of unplanned urbanization, and because of increasing security issues, reluctantly and desperately let their children spend time and play games online. However, those games are not innocent. Most parents state that their children cheer up during playtime; feel sad and start to cry when they lose the game; experience cramps out of excitement and adrenalin in their bodies; adopt highly serious manners, and "pretend" isolating themselves from the world outside during playtime. The most significant sociological problem is that children do not go out, talk to anyone, and engage in any communication even with their relatives living in the same house because they get the illusion that they have already been socialized in cyberspaces; also it harms the notion of family which is the cornerstone of society. One of the most significant psychological problems is that children who stick themselves on computer monitors in a room gradually become isolated, alienated, and adopt an excessive ambition and violence tendency, and demonstrate emotional insufficiencies, as well as the sense of incapability in parallel with the loss of success in real life. This study assesses digital game addiction in the light of the responses to the questions addressed to 350 students consisting of 1st, 2nd, 3rd, and 4th grades in some primary schools in Istanbul who play a game called ROBLOX and 245 family members.

Keywords: digital games, game addiction, digital natives, internet addiction, Roblox

Introduction

Today, the "Technology Acceptance Model" is a model used for analyzing behavior in digital media. According to the model, proposed by Fred Davis in 1989, all the impacts that external factors have on behavior depends on usefulness and ease of use (Yengin, 2014: 85–86).

While there are some who think that the Internet has liberated and individuated people, there are also those who say it has isolated people and made them more easily controllable within the system. Hundreds of millions of people are, each minute, creating and consuming an untold amount of digital content in an online world that is not truly bound by terrestrial laws (Schmidt ve Cohen, 2013: 11–12).

Palm-sized tablets and smartphones with the Internet connection are now one of the biggest addictions for everyone, young and old alike. This addiction has enabled individuals to appear to be stronger and more independent within the current system; however, it has, in fact, made them more controllable and trackable in a way. According to Sussman (2003: 33), communication technologies and social media are created in such a way in terms of the economic structure that they reinforce the power of the rich and the powerful, and while they manufacture users' consents, they basically aim at maintaining the continuity of the global capital.

The word "digital" which is a magical word of today's world appears in various areas from social life to business life and education to entertainment and represents the generation of the children of our era. This new generation is an effective user of this digital media they were born into, and yet they are also exposed to the negative effects resulting from intense arguments within the digital media. Digital game addiction is a leading negative effect.

The biggest problem of today's children is that they cannot go outside and play in a comfortable and safe way. Inadequacy of playgrounds and increasing security problems resulting from conurbation and dense housing play important roles in this issue. Moreover, parents give consent to their children to spend time on the internet due to the time issue of the metropolitan life. Digital games that alienate children from their families, friends, and social life by isolating them from real life may reach very dangerous levels when played without strict controls and time limitations of parents.

In this study, digital game addiction is evaluated in the light of the answers to the questions directed to 350 students aged 7–11 playing ROBLOX and 245 family members. The objective is to contribute to revealing the social and psychological aspects of the problems caused by playing digital games at an extreme level. The study also looks for suggestions for solving these problems.

Digital Natives and Internet

In studies carried out in parallel with the speed and continuity of technological developments, users are discussed under such conceptual names as "digital native", "digital hybrid", and "digital immigrant". People born in and after the year 1980 are called digital natives (Prensky, 2001: 1–6). Those who were born between the years 1970 and 1999 and use both printed and digital sources are labeled as digital hybrids. Also, those who teach digital natives, grown up with digital media and also generally called the "net generation" are called digital immigrants (Yıldız, 2012: 820–823).

In Turkey, the generation called digital hybrid coincides with the start of the computerization process. According to the 2009–2011 data of the Turkish

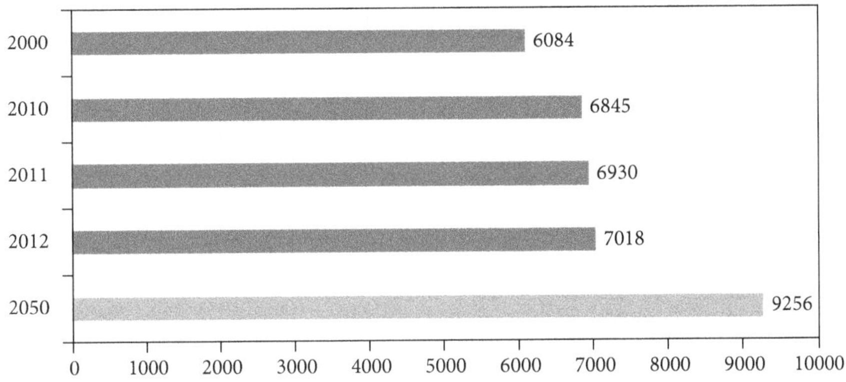

Fig. 1: The Distribution of Internet Use among the World's Population (Yurdakul et al., 2013: 884).

Statistical Institute (TÜİK), the use of the Internet, in parallel with technological developments, increased during the 2000s. Those born in this period fell directly in the embrace of technology.

As can be understood from the figure above, there is an increase in the use of the Internet between the years 2000 and 2012 around the world. "*According to the data published in June 2012, the number of Internet users in Turkey is 36,455,000*" (Yurdakul et al., 2013: 884).

According to the data published in August 2013 by TÜİK, children get acquainted with computer, mobile phone and internet at a very early age. "*Among computer users aged 6–15 in Turkey, the average age to start using a computer is 8, and the average age to start using the Internet is 9. While 24.4 % of children aged 6–15 have their own computers, 13.1 % of them have mobile phones, and 2.9 % of them have game consoles. 60.5 % of the children use computer, 50.8 % use internet and 24.3 % use mobile phone. As for the average weekly time spent using the Internet by children aged 6–15, 38.2 % of them spend about 2 hours online; 47.4 % spend 2 to 10 hours; 11.8 % spend 11 to 24 hours, and 2.6 % spend over 24 hours. 84.8 % of children aged 6–15 use the Internet to do homework and research; 79.5 % of them use it to play games; 56.7 % use it to search for information, and 53.5 % use it to access social media networks. Among children aged 6–15, the average age to start using a mobile phone is 10; its foremost intended use is to call someone, with a percentage of 92.8 %, and the other uses are to play games (66.8 %), to send text-messages (65.4 %) and to use the Internet (30.7 %). 80 % of*

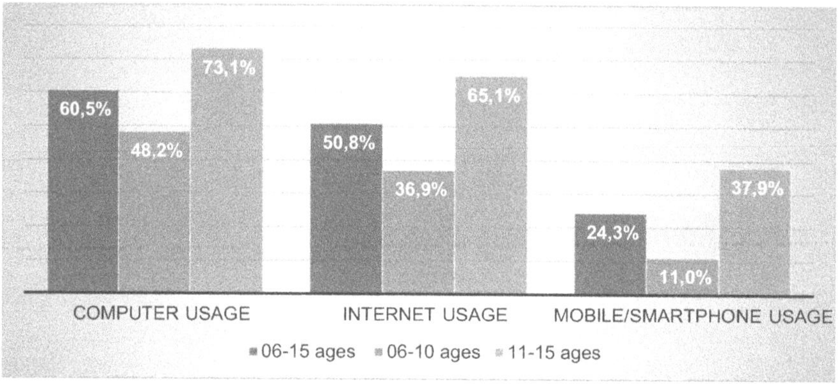

Fig. 2: Internet Usage among Young Population (Türkiye İstatistik Kurumu [TÜİK], 2013).

children aged 6–10 who use a mobile phone play games on their mobiles" (Türkiye İstatistik Kurumu [TÜİK], 2013).

The results of the 2009 EU Kids Online Survey provides important data on the place of the Internet in children's lives. "*Across Europe, one third of 9–10-year-olds use the Internet daily, and this rises to 80 % among 15–16-year-olds*". The same study indicates that the most common location of the internet use is home and that 83 % of children aged 9–16 go online to play games (London School of Economics and Political Science, 2009).

The same survey includes parents, as well, and there are some striking findings. "*70 % of parents talk to their children about what they do on the internet and 50 % stay nearby when the child is online and 12,5 % to do parental control to their children. Over half of parents also take over positive steps such as suggesting how to behave towards others online (56 %) and talking about things that might bother the child (52 %), and a third have helped their child when something arose in the past (36 %). Parents also restrict children's disclosure of personal information (85 %), downloading (63 %) and uploading (57 %). One in two parents monitors their child's internet use (after use)*" (London School of Economics and Political Science, 2009).

The Relationship between Children and Digital Games

Although how, when and where people play games change from age to age, play is a phenomenon which has been present since the existence of human beings.

"Play is man's first art", says Jean-Paul Sartre, and Ferdinand Stangel defines play as the reinforcement and completion of life. According to Huizinga, "*Culture arises in the form of play that is played from the very beginning. If the scope of our actions is deeply analysed, we can call all human activity 'play'.*" (Huizinga, 1995: 27). According to Huizinga, play is freedom, and it can be reproduced. Play is related to order; playing is attractive and a serious act (Huizinga, 1995, 24).

Eric Berne defines game as "*an ongoing series of complementary ulterior transactions progressing to a well-defined, predictable outcome*" (Berne, 1964: 44). According to Caillois, a game is an activity which is essentially free, separate, uncertain, unproductive, governed by rules and make-believe (Caillois, 2001: 10–11).

Traditional games are based on interpersonal communication, physicality and creativity. However, the rapid development and change of technology has transformed traditional games into digital games (Yengin, 2012: 107–111). In other words, today, video games, electronic games, computer games, console games, mobile games, etc. which are gathered under the digital name by moving away from the traditional structure are at the forefront. In this context, digital game is an "*individual communication medium which has such features as digitalness, interactivity, virtuality, variability and modularity and which incorporates these features in the act of playing itself. These media include and keep the concepts and features described as old or conventional*" (Binark et al., 2009: 45). Especially the "addiction" to digital games on tablets and smartphones—which children do not want to put down— is one of the problems of today that are being discussed and that need resolving.

Technological innovations that renew and update themselves every day and digital gaming within this context also include elements of addiction and addictiveness particularly for children. According to Türk Dil Kurumu, the word "addict" is defined as "*a person who is dependent on the desire, help or power of another thing, who lacks independence and freedom, and who is physically or spiritually extremely dependent on a person or thing*" (Türk Dil Kurumu, 2018). As Kırık (2013: 87) points out there are two aspects of addiction as substance addiction and behavioral addiction. Here, it is possible to address the phenomenon as substance addiction if smartphones and tablets are considered substances, and as behavioral addiction if it is viewed as a situation where the person cannot take him/herself from playing games. Young has identified eight items for individuals to be identified as addicted to the Internet and stated that a dependency status has been formed if five of these eight items are met:

1. *Constantly thinking about the Internet and the activities done thereof,*
2. *Being in need of using more Internet with a growing desire, thinking that it is joyful,*

3. *Failure to control or reduce Internet usage,*
4. *Experiencing anger, discomfort when attempting to reduce Internet usage,*
5. *Staying on the Internet more than it was planned at the outset,*
6. *Having problems with family, friends, school, job, career etc. due to excessive use of the Internet,*
7. *Lying to others about the duration of staying on the Internet,*
8. *Viewing the internet as an escape gate to get away from negative emotions and thoughts, that is, as a way of escaping from the reality* (Şakiroğlu and Akyol, 2018: 35–36).

Many parents state that while playing games, their children crow when they win, get frustrated and start to cry when they lose, have contractions in their bodies due to excitement and adrenaline, or have very serious manners, but in fact, they get away from the real world and "pretend" during the game. In this context, it can be argued that children's inner and outer worlds are under intense influence, and that children break loose from the outside world and develop peculiar lives for themselves in a different world which is often difficult to control for their parents. These forms of expression concur with McLuhan's definition of "*the medium is the message, and it's the mass media that shape the world*"(McLuhan, 2001: 201). Each technological medium which developed and changed in the context of technological developments has transformed into a common language through which children communicate with and send messages to each other. The brands and features of the mobile phone, tablet or computer they use have the characteristics of a message even before they start to utilize them in the gaming environment.

"*The acquisition of playing games is realized as sub-genres in the form of console games, PC games and on-line games in the virtual space. In Level computer game magazine which is extensively followed today in the field of computer games, these digital games are classified as Network, Action, Adventure, Motorsports and Race, Role Playing/Animation, Simulation, Sports and Strategy games according to their thematic and technological characteristics*" (Gürcan et al., 2008: 4). Online games, by definition, can be played both individually, and interactively with multiple people simultaneously. Individuals can play games and communicate with each other simultaneously, although they are at different locations in the world. Individuals become even more occupied with the game they play with the characters they create. Because individuals consider themselves in a kind of socialization, they might spend excessive time, even in an uncontrolled way at times, in these games.

It is possible to make assessments about the games both positively and negatively. Games have positive impacts, especially on children, on several domains such as socialization, entertainment, learning, learning/developing a foreign language, creativity, achievement, control and coordination of multiple tasks at the same time, problem-solving and strategy development and being part of the team. "*Scientists in NASA evaluate the impacts of computer games, especially on children with hyperactivity and attention deficit; the results of their research shows that children learn concentration that they experience the feeling of control and superiority and, as a consequence, that the brain generates high frequency waves and learns to be careful thanks to computer games*" (Tarhan and Nurmedov, 2017: 59). Despite the positive reviews, there are sociological, psychological and physiologic problems that arise because digital games cause addiction.

The major sociological problems are that children do not go out because they think they are socialized in the virtual domain, that they do not speak to anyone, not even to their first-degree relatives with whom they live in the same house, and the degeneration of the family, which is the keystone of the society, as a consequence of these negative developments. The most important psychological problems can be summarized as the loneliness of children who isolate themselves in a room experiencing alienation, inclination to extreme ambition and violence, emotional inadequacies, etc. In a study by Holman *et al.*, "*children who use the Internet extensively and spend most of their times with computer games were found to have low self-esteem, demonstrate high levels of social anxiety and aggressive behaviors and that their social development was significantly diminished*"(Holman et al., 2005: 1–6). The primary physiological problems arising from playing these games excessively are, according to a report by AMATEM (Alcohol Drug Addiction Treatment): the wrist syndrome, stiffness in the neck muscles, decreased sleep hours, fatigue in the eyes, obesity, circulatory system disorders, etc. Gentile, Anderson and Buckley who conduct studies on the digital gaming environment "*reveal in their study on the impacts of video games on children the harms of violence extant in video games with the general aggression model and state that it has negative impacts especially on children's academic achievement and school performance*" (Anderson et al., 2007: 90), The most effective way to overcome these problems is parents' setting role models to develop solutions regarding the use of the internet, computers, tablets, smart phones and games that are inevitable necessities of this age, rather than imposing punishments, sanctions or reprimand. "*Especially mobile technology has caused the physical and virtual universes to intermingle*" (Varna, 2013: 219). It is known that parents can sustain the roles they assume every time and everywhere as a result of this intermingling. In simpler words, while the business life stayed at the workplace in the past, now it can be maintained anytime in any place due to mobile technologies. Another or father who is a manager or a worker at the workplace can sustain their same roles as a manager or worker at home, which demonstrates the care and time stolen from children. Possible problems can be avoided if the parents, rather than retreating a corner with their smartphones, tablets or PCs when they are home, communicate with their children through proper timing within the familial environment, play games with them, determine the studying times for children accurately, appropriately plan when children can play digital games on the internet and abide by this planning themselves too.

> *"According to the Global Children and Gaming Study carried out by OMO (Unilever's Detergent Brand) in 12 countries on 12,000 parents in 2016, 56 % of children play less than one hour in the open air per day on average and 19 % of them play less than 30 minutes. This is even less than the minimum duration of staying in the open air recommended by the Office of the UN High Commissioner for Human Rights regarding prisoners"* (Dışarı çıkmayan çocuklar, n.d.).

Roblox as the New Online Venue for Digital Natives

In digital games, children can play what they want, communicate with anyone and do whatever they want to through the avatars (virtual identities) they create for themselves. As Giddens notes, "*the people in cyberspace are no longer 'people' but messages on each other's screens*" (2001: 42). In this context, children have the freedom of speaking and behaving as they want without disclosing their real identities. This situation, which seems to be freedom, is in fact an escape of the individual from his/her own reality to the virtual world that he/she has created for various reasons. This world, which is individual by any aspect, also builds a virtual society for itself and creates a virtual socialization. Children's familial sharing have been restricted as a result of shifting from large family structures to nuclear families, together with women's assuming more effective roles in the family structure and the living conditions deteriorated by the capitalist system due to industrialization. The first source of learning for the child is the family. Within this context, "*family is the institution in which the foundations of the connection of individuals with the society is built. The individual, first of all, learns socialization with his/her behaviors in the family and then, use this notion to enlarge/regulate his/her milieu*" (Karakoç, 2013: 212). The child who becomes isolated in the family gets a lot of knowledge and experience from this virtual environment by being exposed to dangers while trying to find arbitrary solutions to loneliness through the digital games he/she plays.

Tab. 1: Gender Distribution of Participants (Parents)

Participants	**Frequency (f)**	**Percentage (%)**
Female	168	68.6
Male	77	31.4
Total	**245**	**100**

In the case study, this digital gaming addiction has been addressed through a survey on 350 students studying at the 1st, 2nd, 3rd and 4th grades of certain elementary schools in Istanbul and 245 family members within the scope of the ROBLOX game. The *ROBLOX game, which was chosen as the case, is an MMOG game targeting 8–18-year old. In the game, users can make their virtual worlds by changing the color and size of blocks in various shapes that other users can enter* (Roblox, 2018). In this study, digital gaming habits of children who are at the ages ranging between 7 and 11 are measured and evaluations are conducted based on information provided by the parents of these children. Moreover, suggestions on digital gaming addiction and its future are presented in line with the findings.

Findings

In the part related to parents, the target population of the survey is mostly women.

According to the information on gender distribution in Tab. 1, 68.6 % of the participants are women, and 31.4 % are men. In the light of this information, it is not wrong to say that women are more interested in this survey, which is closely related to child development.

It is seen that 48.2 % of the participants are 40–44 years old, and 30.6 % are 35–39 years old. 73.5 % have bachelor's degree, and 26.5 % have PhD and master's degree. Another detail is that 43.7 % of the participants are self-employed, and 40.8 % are wage-earners.

While 53.1 % of the participants say that their child goes online after school to play games for 1–3 hours, 31.4 % say that this duration is less than an hour.

As for the device the child uses to go online, the percentage for tablet use is 55.5 %, the one for smartphone use is 22.4 %, and that for computer use is 18.4 %. Of the families, 83.3 % state that their child goes online after school to play games.

67.3 % of the parents state that their child plays Roblox. While 20.4 % say that their child plays Minecraft, 3.3 % (8 parents) say that their child "does not

Tab. 2: Demographics of Participants

Groups	Frequency (f)	Percentage (%)
Age		
20–24	0	0
25–29	0	0
30–34	24	9.8
35–39	75	30.7
40–44	118	48.2
45–49	20	8.2
50–54	8	3.3
55 and over	0	0
Level of Education		
Primary education	0	0
Secondary education	0	0
Associate degree	0	0
Bachelor's degree	180	735
Master's degree and PhD	65	26.5
Profession		
Student	0	0
Self-employed	107	43.7
Wage-earner	100	40.8
Unemployed	20	8.2
Other	18	7.3

play games", a remarkable fact. It is not wrong to point out that almost all of the participants' children spend time online playing digital games.

At a high rate of 64.1 %, parents stated that their children did not communicate with them while they were playing digital games, they did not answer any question or even give any reaction to any statement. At a rate of 29.8 %, they also stated that their children seemed stressful to them.

The percentage of parents who stated that the behaviors they observed in their children after playing digital games were aggressive, conditioning for behaving as they desire, and shouting is 89 %. The percentage of those who think that their children are addicted to games is 64.9 %, while the percentage of those who think the contrary is 35.1 %.

> *"94 % of parents in Turkey think that children who do not have the opportunity to play games outdoors will have difficulty in learning, while 70 % believe that their children do*

Tab. 3: Information on Parents' Observations on Their Children's Internet Use

Groups	Frequency (f)	Percentage (%)
Duration of the time the child spends playing online games after school or during holidays		
Less than 1 hour	77	31.4
1–3 hours	130	53.1
Over 3 hours	30	12.2
None	8	3.3
The device the child uses to go online		
Television	8	3.3
Computer	45	18.4
Laptop	1	0.4
Tablet	136	55.5
Smartphones	55	22.4
What the child does during his/her time on the Internet after school?		
Research	12	16.7
Play games	60	83.3
The game the child plays		
Roblox	165	67.3
Minecraft	50	20.4
Grand Theft	0	0
Other	22	9
Not playing	8	3.3

> *not have sufficient opportunity to play outside. 59 % of the parents want their children to have a better balance in indoor and outdoor games. 57 % of the parents in Turkey believe that their children have fewer opportunities to play games compared to their own childhood"* (Dışarı çıkmayan çocuklar, n.d.).

92.2 % of the parents stated that they had a regular control over their children's use of the internet, 66.9 % of them stated that they used a security lock to limit their children's use of the internet. The parents participating in the research were asked "What do you think about your child's spending time on the internet and on digital games?" They thought that the use of internet was inevitable as a necessity of the age, but it was necessary to check and control the children's use of the internet, their interest in digital games and the time they spend on these.

Tab. 4: Parents' Observations on Their Children's Playing Digital Games

Groups	Frequency (f)	Percentage (%)
How the child behaves while playing digital games?		
Not communicating	157	64.1
Being aggressive	10	4.1
Being stressful	73	29.8
Other	5	2
How the child behaves after playing digital games?		
Being aggressive, İmposing conditions before doing what you want them to do, shouting	218	89
Throwing things	0	0
Other	27	11
What you think about your child's being a "game addict"?		
Yes, I think.	159	64.9
No, I don't think.	86	35.1

Tab. 5: Information on Parents' Control of Internet Use and Safety Lock

Groups	Frequency (f)	Percentage (%)
Do you always control your child's internet use?		
Yes, I do.	226	92.2
No, I don't.	19	7.8
Do you use safety lock on your child's computer?		
Yes, I do.	164	66.9
No, I don't.	81	33.1

Most of the children are 8 years (41.7 %) and 9 years (37.7 %) old. Majority of the children are fourth grade (44 %) and third grade (40%).

Whereas 334 children (95.4 %) stated that they were playing games, 16 children (4.6 %) stated that they were not. They mostly play Roblox (61.1 %). 68.3 % of the children were playing games for 1 to 3 hours and 19.1 % of them were playing games for less than 1 hour. While 64.3 % stated that they were playing

Tab. 6: Demographics of Participants (Children)

Groups	Frequency (f)	Percentage (%)
Gender		
Female	161	46
Male	189	54
Total:	**350**	**100**
Age		
06	0	0
07	36	10.3
08	146	41.7
09	132	37.7
10	36	10.3
Level of education		
1.grade	0	0
2.grade	56	16
3.grade	140	40
4.grade	154	44

digital games on the internet every day, only 16 (4.5 %) of them were not playing games. Most of the children (60.6 %) uses tablets to play digital games.

56 % of the children indicated that they play a certain digital game because of the "content". On the other hand, 23.4 % of them were playing games upon a friend's advice. While 52.6 % of the children were not playing games one after another, 42.8 % of them stated just the opposite. A large proportion of the children (74.6 %) stated that they spent time on the internet after school or on holidays.

41.7 % of the children stated that they feel excited when playing games and 40 % of them have fun. Playing outside is a leading favorite activity by 54.6 % compared to playing digital games on the internet. This is followed by "meeting friends", with a rate of 18.6 % and "playing games with the family", with a rate of 13.1 %. The children were asked whether they felt tired while playing digital games. 79.4 % of the children responded that they felt tired.

The children were asked whether they got angry with their parents when they told them to give a break to the digital game. 79.4 % of the children stated that they got angry. A large proportion of the children (73.3 %) reported that they did not feel the desire to play digital games when they were outside. Indeed, a

Tab. 7: Children's Preferences Regarding Digital Gaming

Groups	Frequency (f)	Percentage (%)
Do you play digital games?		
Yes, I play games.	334	95.4
No, I don't play games.	16	4.6
What digital games do you play?		
Roblox	214	61.1
Minecraft	55	15.7
Grand Theft	0	0
Other	65	18.6
Not playing	16	4.6
How many hours a day do you play digital games?		
Less than 1 hour	67	19.1
1–3 hours	239	68.3
Over 3 hours	28	8
Not playing	16	4.6
How many days per week do you play games?		
1–2 days	34	9.7
3–4 days	52	14.9
5–6 days	23	6.6
Every day	225	64.3
Not playing	16	4.5
What device do you prefer to play games?		
Computer	32	9.1
Laptop	11	3.1
Tablet	212	60.6
Smartphones	79	22.6
Not playing	16	4.6

large proportion of the children (78.6 %) preferred playing with friends outside to playing digital games.

The children were asked an open-ended question to find out why they wanted to play digital games on the internet. Analyses of the answers of girls showed that 59 % of them played games as they were enjoyable, 21.7 % of them played games not to feel bored as they had nothing else to do and 11.2 % of them played games to spend their time when their parents showed no interest in them. The answer of an 8-year-old girl was particularly interesting: "My

Tab. 8: Children's Reasons for Playing Digital Games

Groups	Frequency (f)	Percentage (%)
Why the child plays the game that he/she loves to play		
Because of its content	196	56
Because of awards	14	4
Upon a friend's recommendation	82	23.4
Because it is a popular game that everyone talks about	42	12
Not playing	16	4.6
Whether the child tends to play different games in a row		
Yes	150	42.8
No	184	52.6
Not playing	16	4.6
What the child does when they go online after school/during holidays		
Research	89	25.4
Play games	261	74.6

mom is not at home when I come home, neither is my father. And my grandmother is only interested in her friends. There is nobody to take care of me, what else can I do other than playing games on the internet?". Analyses of the answers of boys to the question which intended to find out why they wanted to play digital games on the internet showed that 77.8 % of them found games enjoyable and they had the chance to virtually meet their friends on the internet and play the game together, 36.9 % of them played digital games to spend their free time and 15.4 % of them stated that they did not know why they played digital games. 8 girls and 8 boys stated that they have never played games.

It was observed that the aspect of "fun" was at the forefront regarding their expectations of children from digital games and boys found digital games enjoyable more than girls. A total of 350 children participated in the research, 189 were boys and 161 were girls. The study shows that there is no significant difference between boys and girls in terms of the interest in digital games. Only 16 out of 350 participants stated that they never played digital games, which reveals out the addiction of today's children to digital games.

Tab. 9: Children's Emotions While Playing Digital Games

Groups	Frequency (f)	Percentage (%)
What do you feel while playing online digital games?		
Happy	22	6.3
Amused	140	40
Excited	146	41.7
Stressful	26	7.4
Not playing	16	4.6
What do you like doing more than playing online digital games?		
Playing outside	191	54.6
Playing with my family	46	13.1
Meeting friends	65	18.6
Chatting with my family	4	1.1
Going to the theatre/cinema	25	7.1
Other	3	0.9
Not playing	16	4.6
Do you feel tired while/after playing digital games?		
Yes, I feel tired.	278	79.4
No, I don't feel tired.	56	16
I don't play games.	16	4.6

Conclusion

It can be argued, within the scope of the study, that most of the children are digital gaming addicts. Although digital gaming seems to have certain advantages in terms of children's time spending, enhancing their imagination and designing aspects, having fun and learning, excessive digital gaming, as a fact that parents hardly acknowledge or perhaps ignore, involves physiologic and physiological dangers. Digital games that isolate, alienate and break children from their families, peers and the social life by taking them apart from the real life, can reach dangerous levels when played in the absence of strict control and time limitations by the parents. The primary measures to protect children from such negative effects of digital gaming include making children allocate the time they spend playing digital games for more useful social activities, making arrangements with respect to game playing times, providing a reminder for children by setting

Tab. 10: Children's Preferences of Digital Games

Groups	Frequency (f)	Percentage (%)
Do you get angry with your parents when they tell you to take a break from playing?		
Yes, I get angry.	278	79.4
No, I don't get angry.	56	16
I don't play games.	16	5.6
Do you want to play digital games even when you are outside?		
Yes, I do want to play digital games even when I'm outside.	77	22.00
No, I don't want to play digital games when I'm outside.	257	73.4
I don't play games.	16	4.6
Do you prefer to play online digital games or play outside with your friends?		
I prefer to play outside with my friends.	275	78.6
I prefer to play online digital games.	75	21.4

the alarm when making the time arrangement, enhancing intra-family communication in a robust way, supporting the children by teaching them to be sensitive in time management, constantly reminding the parents about the consciousness that they need to be role models in the use of technological devices, monitoring children's internet usage, and creating environments in which children can socialize in natural ways.

As identified in the study, the vast majority of families stated that their children played games for 1 to 3 hours a day, they could not take back the smartphones and tablets and other similar devices from their children and felt uncomfortable about their children's spending time playing digital games on these devices; however, they also stated that they do not consider playing digital games for three straight hours to be addiction for children who are 7–10 years old. It can be claimed that parents may have difficulty in expressing their real opinions in the study although the survey was conducted totally unanimously. Especially, behaviors such as children's not communicating with their parents and surroundings during the games, behaving aggressively, imposing conditions to fulfill what their parents ask them to do and shouting after the game are among the main complaints of the families. Despite all of these reactions, a great majority, 64.9 %, of the parents who participated in the survey, do not consider their children “Internet or gaming addicts”. All parents responded to the open-ended question stating that controlled Internet and digital gaming would be beneficial for children.

Children’s answers to the survey was in parallel with their parents. They stated that they spend time on the Internet playing digital games for 1–3 hours a day, every day. 63.7 % of the children indicated that they were tired when they played digital games, and 79.4 % of them stated that they got angry at their parents when they told them that they had to take a break from playing games. The responses of female students to the open-ended question about why they play digital games on the Internet are as follows: because they find it enjoyable, for not getting bored and for not having anyone to take care of them at home, respectively in terms of frequencies. Responses of the male students to the same question are as follows: for they find it enjoyable, for not getting bored in their spare times and that they do not know why they play, still respectively in terms of frequencies.

In IT society any sorts of data and information can be collected, classified, processed and transferred rapidly and effectively People can access any kind of data easily wherever and whenever they want, and they can also be a source in the dissemination of new data and information. Digitization in the communication environment manifests the necessity of stricter controls and supervision especially in the usage domains of children. Digital games, that are enjoyed by children, bear many dangers for children while presenting a colorful virtual world to them. These threats are not only related to the contents of digital games with violence, sexuality, etc. but also to the sociological, psychological and physiological diseases arising from “the desire for untimely / unlimited playing” in relation to the charm of digital games. In particular, several problems such as aggressive behaviors, weight gain caused by inactivity, circulatory disorders, skeletal structure disorders, self-isolation, alienation, escaping from socializing that are observed in children during or after playing digital games create big problems for the family as well as children.

The subjects children question changes in parallel with the development of communication technologies. The most addictive fruit of the technology children of the millennium age were born into is the digital games. This indicates that nesting the concepts of game and homework is inevitable. It is neither possible to hinder the innovations brought about by time and technology, nor would it be a solution to impose strict prohibitions. For this reason, allowing children to have this catharsis by having them think of their classes like a leisure time activity, developing an education approach by focusing on learning-by-playing methods with the aim of combining children’s skills of imagination, designing, IT and developing different perspectives with games can make a certain amelioration if cannot completely eliminate the digital game addiction problem. Education and seminars that teach children that the digital world and its advantages should be used without letting them prevail their significant life activities an important part of the curricula would be an important step to be taken regarding this subject matter.

When they are used promptly and effectively, reaching out to the imaginary world of children, the Internet and digital games have a potential to contribute to their personal and mental development by protecting them from the bad effects of this imaginary world. As a matter of fact, it is possible to transform digital games into a useful activity and means of entertainment for children with the monitoring of parents and teachers. In this context, it will not be wrong to use Huizinga's phrase "Cta est fabula" (game over) for digital games, of which we know the dangerous aspects and how to take them under control (Yalım, 2013).

Bibliography

Akyol, P. C. & Şakiroğlu, M. (2018). Çocukları Sanal Dünyada(n) Koruma Kılavuzu. İstanbul: Hayykitap.

Anderson, C., Gentile, D. & Buckley, K. (2007). Violent Video Game Effects on Children and Adolescents: Theory, Research, and Public Policy. Oxford: Oxford University Press.

Berne, E. (1964). Games People Play: The Psychology of Human Relationship. London: Penguin Books.

Binark, M., Bayraktutan-Sütçü, G. & Fidaner, I. B. (2009). Dijital Oyun Rehberi: Oyun Tasarımı, Türler ve Oyuncu. İstanbul: Kalkedon Yayınları.

Büyükaslan, A. & Kırık, M. A. (2013). Sosyal Medya Araştırmaları 1-Sosyalleşen Birey, Kırık, M. A. "Gelişen Web Teknolojileri ve Sosyal Medya Bağımlılığı". Konya: Çizgi Kitabevi.

Caillois, R. (2001). Man, Play and Game. Illınois: University of Illinois Press.

Dışarı çıkmayan çocuklar: Rakamlarla günümüz çocuklarının sokakla imtihanı. (n.d.). Retrieved from http://www.hurriyet.com.tr/kesfet/disari-cikmayan-cocuklar-rakamlarla-gunumuz-cocuklarinin-sokakla-imtihani-40801751 on 2 May 2018

Giddens, A. (2001). Sociology, 4th ed. Oxford, Polity Press.

Gürcan, A., Özhan, S. & Uslu, R. (2008). Dijital Oyunlar ve Çocuklar Üzerindeki Etkileri. Ankara: T.C. Başbakanlık Aile ve Sosyal Araştırmalar Genel Müdürlüğü.

Holman, J. P., Hansen, C. E., Cochian, M. E., Lindsey, C. R. (2005). Liar, Liar: Internet Faking but not Frequency of Use Affect Social Skills, Self-Esteem, Social Anxiety, and Aggression, Cyberpsychology & Behaviour, 8(1), 1–6.

Huizinga, J. (1995). Homo Ludens Oyunun Toplumsal İşlevi Üzerine Bir Deneme (M.A. Kılıçbay, Trans.). İstanbul: Ayrıntı Yayınları.

Huizinga, J. (2006). Oyunun Toplumsal İşlevi Üzerine Bir Deneme "Homo Ludens". İstanbul: Ayrıntı Yayınları.

Karakoç, E. (2013). Toplumsal Dönüşüm Bağlamında Sosyal Medya ve Değişen Aile Kavramı. In A. Büyükaslan & A.M. Kırık (Eds.), Sosyal Medya Araştırmaları 1 Sosyalleşen Birey (pp. 207–224). Konya: Çizgi Kitabevi Yayınları.

Kırık, A. M. (2013). Gelişen Web Teknolojileri ve Sosyal Medya Bağımlılığı Sosyalleşen Birey. In A. Büyükaslan & A.M. Kırık, (Eds.), Sosyal Medya Araştırmaları 1 (pp. 69–102). Konya: Çizgi Yayınevi.

London School of Economics and Political Science. (2009). Avrupa Çevrim İçi Çocuklar Projesi Özet Bulguları, Retrieved from http://www.lse.ac.uk/media@lse/research/EUKidsOnline/EU%20Kids%20II%20(2009-11)/EUKidsExecSummary/TurkeyExecSum.pdfon 18 April 2018

McLuhan, M. (2001). Global Köy. İstanbul: Scala Yayıncılık.

Prensky, M. (2001). Digital Natives, Digital Immigrants. On the Horizon, 9(5), 1–6. Retrieved from https://www.emeraldinsight.com/doi/pdfplus/10.1108/10748120110424816.

Roblox. (2018). Retrieved May 3, 2018, from Wikizero: http://www.wikizero.net/index.php?q=aHR0cHM6Ly90ci53aWtpcGVkaWEub3JnL3dpa2kvUm9ibG94.

Schmidt, E., & Cohen, J. (2014). The New Digital Age: Transforming Nations, Businesses and Our Lives. USA: Vintage.

Sussman, G. (2003). Informational Technology and Transnational Networks: A World Systems Approach. In L. Artz & Y. R. Kamalipour (Eds.), The Globalization of Corporate Media Hegemony (pp. 33–53). New York: State University of New York Press.

Tarhan, N. & Nurmedov, S. (2017). Bağımlılık Sanal veya Gerçek. İstanbul: Timaş Yayınları.

Türk Dil Kurumu. (2018). Retrieved from http://www.tdk.gov.tr/index.php?option=com_gts&arama=gts&guid=TDK.GTS.5b0e99f4eae461.42422244-12.04.2018 on 12 April 2018.

Türkiye İstatistik Kurumu. (2013, August 22). 06–15 Yaş Grubu Çocuklarda Bilişim Teknolojileri Kullanımı Ve Medya. Retrieved from http://www.tuik.gov.tr/PdfGetir.do?id=15866 on 9 April 2018.

Varnalı, K. (2013). Dijital Tutulma Pazarlama İletişimi ve İnsan. İstanbul: MediaCat.

Yalım. (2013, November 6). Oyun Oynayan İnsan ve Huizinga [blogpost]. Retrieved from http://www.hulyayalim.com/oyun-oynayan-insan-ve-huizinga/. on 4 June 2018

Yengin, D. (2012). Dijital Oyunlarda Şiddet. İstanbul: Beta.

Yengin, D. (2014). Yeni Medya ve Dokunmatik Toplum. İstanbul: Derin Yayınları.

Yıldız, K. A. (2012). Dijital Yerliler Gerçekten Yerli mi Yoksa Dijital Melez mi? International Journal of Social Science, 5(7), 819–833. Retrieved from https://www.academia.edu/7391948/DİJİTAL_YERLİLER_GERÇEKTEN_YERLİ_Mİ_YOKSA_DİJİTAL_MELEZ_Mİ_ARE_DIGITAL_NATIVES_REALLY_NATIVES_OR_DIGITAL_HYBRIDS?auto=download. on 13 May 2018.

Yurdakul, I. K., Dönmez, O., Yaman, F. & Odabaşı, H. F. (2013). Dijital Ebeveynlik ve Değişen Roller. Gaziantep University Journal of Social Science, 12(4), 883–896. Retrieved from http://dergipark.gov.tr/download/article-file/223235 on 20 May 2018.

Nur Emine Koç

Binge Watching

Abstract: This chapter points out danger waiting us together with the development of technology, which is "binge watching" used to refer to watching episodes of series one after another. With the purpose of revealing the underlying reasons of binge watching and the effects of it on watchers, the study has examined why the watchers prefer to watch the digital platform series they actively watch, which series are preferred by the watchers displaying binge watching behavior, and what are the permanent effects of that binge watching on those watchers. Addictive digital platform series whose numbers are gradually increasing isolate watchers from the real life, sometimes taking the whole day of the watchers. Binge watching, which could cause several health problems, such as heart disease, blood pressure disorders, obesity, and cancer as a result of excessive immobility, has now become an issue in Turkey, too. Considering the proliferation of digital platforms and the habits of the internet use, especially of the young population, it has been determined that the series and movies market will maintain its existence on digital platforms mostly, and that binge watching behavior will become widespread. On such a significant issue, a focus group study has been conducted through the individuals who watch the series on Netflix, Puhu TV, BluTV, and dizimag5.co, which is a foreign series digital platform, and some striking results have been obtained.

Keywords: binge watching, digital serials, TV serials, digital addiction

Introduction

In today's world, individuals have accepted and internalized the television world just like people in *Truman Show* and animals in George Orwell's "Animal Farm" and people in George Orwell's "1984". Television, which has been the most popular communication medium since its invention, has showed people things that they have never owned or will never own, and made connections between people, and the characters and incidents to which they feel close. This connection influences the audience just like family members influence their child (Gerbner, 2002: 81). A television, which is left on, is sometimes enough. People are unaware that a television left on affects them. People feel like something is missing, when there is no sound coming from the TV, thus TV is left on even though they do not watch it. In today's media, this feeling is not specific for only television. Rapid development of the digital media and technology has changed audience's focus by replacing traditional TV shows and TV series.

People do not have much knowledge about using these technological devices as a result of its development in a dramatic speed. Moreover, they do not care about how to use these devices. An individual buys and uses devices, machines, and phones that s/he does not know how they work, and s/he does not think about their harms but just their need at that very moment. At this point, television and consumption correlation intersects as the individual places the product, which is an attraction center, at the center of his/her life (Postman, 2014: 101). In Baudrillard's words in the high-speed postmodern world, an individual's need is shaped by the power of the media as s/he does not have time to think about his/her needs (Baudrillard, 2010: 60). The audience is consumer now. The motto "Buy, consume and buy other things" is available not only for goods but also for media shows as consumption rushes as fast as life. The audience, which learns from the media what to consume and how to consume it, experiences love, hate, and any other feelings with the motto "Buy, consume and buy other things". The individual is unaware of the fact that his/her needs are limited to the suggestions proposed by the media. S/he chooses simulation life (which is not reached in real life) in Matrix and to be powerful, rich, and famous (which is not possible in real life) like Cypher[1], who postpones responsibilities and wants to run away from the reality of life as virtual struggle is not enough for the successes in real life. As a result, the audience, which prioritizes pleasure need in Huxley's "Brave New World", stays in happy virtual world and is always ready to consume via media.

Media is the most important factor, which makes consumption constant. TV series sector maintains its popularity both in the USA and in Turkey. Especially new trend on digital media platforms is TV shows which can be watched online. They offer a freer environment without advertisements and censors. However, this freedom becomes an addiction as a result of the unreasonable duration time of TV series. TV series on digital media causes illnesses just like online games which fill up teenager's free time (Fontaine, 2013: 115). Digital platforms, which are similar to the video market of the 80s and 90s, build an audience, which does not detach from television as a result of watching all episodes successively and

---

1 Cypher is a character from the movie Matrix who betrays people deliberately by collaborating with the robots. He aims to go back to the fantasy world with this collaboration despite he comes to real world by escaping from the robots and Matrix (which is a computer based unreal dream jail where people are slept by the robots). He denies the cold and poor side of the real world the situation of being face-to-face with the fear of death and war all the time. In the movie, this character is also a reference to the Judas, who betrayed Jesus.

competes with each other to finish all seasons. Watching TV series on digital media platforms without time limitations and addiction to consume all seasons is called binge watching (Gay, 2013). Binge watching, which freezes time and mind, is one of the striking examples for resetting thoughts and postponing life by running away from the responsibilities.

The aim of this research is to unfold the digital addiction of our era, "binge watching" (watching in rapid succession) with its reasons and harms. This study seeks to research questions such as why the target audience prefers the shows they watch, which shows they tend to follow, and any possible permanent damage inflicted on the viewer by this digital addiction. Nowadays, there are numerous TV shows provided by digital platforms with ever-increasing number of viewers. Such addicting TV shows could even lead to problems where the individuals start spending their whole day at home, losing their grip over the life outside. Leading to various health problems such as heart problems, tension, obesity and cancer; binge watching is an ever-increasing addiction in Turkey. The most popular platforms in Turkey like Netflix, PuhuTV, BluTV and dizimag5.co, and their most watched shows will be compared to their American equivalents, and the study will discuss viewer's interactions with such shows and the motives for making them available for the viewer. The reason for this discussion is to reveal the attitude of the inspected target audience, aged 19 to 29 and 30 to 39, towards the TV shows and to determine the importance and influence of such shows in their lives. The reason for focusing on two different age groups is in order to discover which age group is more likely to watch and fall under such TV show's influence.

Binge Watching

Television is one of the most striking actors in history, which caused socio-economic and sociocultural changes. With the introduction of television into households, the cultural codes have changed; moreover, it even started to shape the attitude of people. According to Gerbner's Cultivation Theory (2002: 76), television has a deep influence on the audience consciously or subconsciously. Furthermore, since TV has the similar effect like a member of the family, it creates views for the audience either involuntarily or purposefully. As the viewer under such psychological influence watches the TV programs such as competition, TV shows, or celebrity news in order to relieve the stress of his/her daily responsibilities, they find themselves misguided into symbolic consumption. In other words, the audience does not watch with the sole purpose of meeting their needs but also enjoys this situation.

Individuals trying to keep pace with the consumption culture have two types of attitude in today's world where the meaning structures are rendered meaningless. People of the 21st century are consuming their time either being overburdened with their work unable to think of anything else or wasting their whole time. In either case, the individual in question consumes everything rapidly just like s/he consumes his/her life, and their principals and ideals are replaced with nonchalance and renunciation. What is more, such renunciation does not lead to penitence (Kristeva, 2017: 32), the consumption continues one way or another. The consumed thing could be an item or time.

Today's consumption is no longer limited to an active interaction with the objects, but it determines our position with the people around us and in the society. As Baudrillard suggests, consumption is not the satisfaction of our natural needs with items and services, it is a global interaction determined by codes and rules (2010: 55). In this global interaction, the individual shapes his/her needs according to the requirements of the consumption society and feels privileged as s/he consumes; however, this makes her/him embrace the consumption society (Baudrillard, 2010: 58).

One of the most important factors that makes consumption continuous is the media. The target audience watching the TV shows might feel happy by means of seeing the life s/he longs for, or s/he might feel unhappy seeing the people as the owners of life s/he might never have. In either case, s/he keeps following these shows. As the audience watches these TV series; they free their minds, isolate themselves from their troubles, and drift apart from the life outside.

Nowadays, the most widely watched programs are TV series. Especially the new trend of digital media platforms is the TV shows which can be watched online. Moreover, the traditional understanding of TV shows are compelled to change by these TV series. With its instant feedback features through comments from viewers, online platforms clearly differentiate the good and bad shows. TV shows on digital platforms, which can also enable easy tracking for the number of viewers, have been actively operative for 10 to 15 years in USA and 8 years in Turkey; however, it started running as an official activity only for the last year. The most prominent ones in Turkey, which also provide a free one-month trial, are Netflix, BluTV, and PuhuTV. PuhuTV offers a free service unlike BluTV and Netflix. In the research, these three platforms and the webpage dizimag5.co has been studied. While TV channels in Turkey still have high ratings, these TV series on aforementioned platforms offer a different experience for the audience and as a result of this the popularity of these platforms has increased rapidly.

Platforms such as Netflix and BluTV, making foreign TV shows available for the audience, have the previous seasons of the TV shows. Turkish viewers who cannot find such TV shows on TV has a chance to watch these shows without any restrictions on the digital platforms. American TV shows with different types of fiction have been attracting a lot of attention and made a place for themselves in the unofficial web pages. After realizing the demand for these shows, Netflix, an online official platform for TV shows, has opened its Turkish branch and brought together Turkish viewers with the foreign shows in January 7, 2016 (Netflix Kurumsal Bilgileri, n.d.). Foreign TV shows with all their seasons available for the audience have been very time consuming, especially for the young audience.

The behavior manifesting itself as some sort of competition among the individuals of consumption society to finish all the episodes of a TV series in 24 hours has not only invaded the minds of younger generation but also the adults. This addiction put forward by the consumption society both in forms of games and TV shows is called binge racing. The term "binge watching", also known as binge-viewing or marathon-viewing, was first added into English vocabulary with Oxford Dictionary in 2013. In Oxford definition "binge-watch" is mentioned as breaking the traditional cycle of watching an episode once a week and a practice/habit/application of freeing the audience and the reason behind the use of this term is the common usage of this term by individuals (Oxford Dictionaries, 2013). The term "Binge watch" has derived from the word "binge". Binge means a period of excessive indulgence in an activity in a short period of time. Having a negative connotation, the word "binge" is also collocated with other words as binge-eat (eating in a rapid succession) or binge-drink (drinking in a rapid succession). In this respect, binge watching made a place for itself in the vocabulary as something which should not be done but also a pleasurable activity when performed (Ramsay, 2013). The term commonly goes as "tıkınmalı izleme" in Turkish (Yengin and Kınay, 2015: 213–257). While watching in rapid succession initially leads to guilt due to its results such as sleeplessness and putting off daily life, it suppresses such negative connotations later, replacing guilt with pleasure. Spreading through bush telegraph and online advertisements like 10 best TV series to watch, and creating an addiction of watching, this habit causes the audience to fully focus on the TV series and losing their grip on reality in the process.

The most obvious behavior which can be observed on the viewers is their complete focus on the screen. Since the viewer, who puts off all his/her needs, sits in a fixed posture, s/he does not work, neither his/her body or brain. Considering the habit of working in a fixed posture for a period of time is harmful, the habit of fixing on the screen numbing one's brain resembles the dystopic country of Oceania in George Orwell's book "1984". Orwell, in his book "1984", pictures a dystopic country based on the dangers of technology.

Every movement of the individuals are tracked by cameras and anyone leaving the boundaries of this country is detected by the cameras and punished (Orwell, 2008: 55). The technology, based on Bentham's prison model (1995), has put the people of Oceania in a permanent "Attention!" status, consequently leading to a maximum level of obedience for the rules set by the government since people had no way of understanding when they were actually being watched. The model of human pictured by Orwell in "1984" is also important in respect with its messages regarding technology. The enormous screens, which are used only when the "Big Brother" demands, include a limited selection of information and messages decided by the country. And this case manipulates the perception of the people of Oceania despite the fact that they are actually prisoners. The protagonist Smith, as much as he tries to resist, cannot prevent his doom as the representative of free thought. This book clearly reflects the use of technology as double-thinking; adopting two opposing ideas. Smith is continuously asked the question "2+2" and tortured until he no longer remembers the correct answer. At the end, when he accepts all the imposed without any objection or reasoning, the torture ends, and he goes back to his life. Smith, who questions nothing, has become an individual devoted to Oceania (Orwell, 2008).

Although Orwell tried to warn countries about the harms of technology to come 40 years later, his thoughts were insufficient. Because what is more dangerous than the dystopic world of Orwell is not the banning of books, being deprived of correct information, to turn into a culture in chains or to suppress emotions to escape punishment and pain. To create a permanent change, it takes plenty of available books and no one in need of reading them, easy access to a wide range of information and no need to learn, and to promote numbness, indifference, and selfishness not by suppression or punishment but by a hedonistic evolution prioritizing pleasure, delight, and indulgence just like it was mentioned in Huxley's "Brave New World" (Huxley, 2007). Although Orwell's world also draws attention to the long-term harmful effects of technology, Huxley's dystopic world is a better fit for the people of the 21st century. The addiction of binge watching is just a proof of how right Huxley was.

As today's viewer desires to indulge himself and fill his/her free time, s/he unconsciously becomes addicted to virtual life and cannot help him/herself not to watch the all the episodes of a TV show, and consequently lose his/her grip over life since s/he cannot do anything else for 24 hours (Jurgensen, 2012: 25–32). Sometimes s/he puts off eating and in other times s/he postpones settling an important task. The viewer experiences a cease in brain functions and loses track of time and location. This situation does not only cause psychological effects, but also leads to physical problems. For instance, a person without physical activity has a higher risk of cardiovascular diseases or cancer compared to one who is physically active. Furthermore, inactivity and excessive eating leads to obesity. The person who loses track of time and location, indulges him/herself in junk food and becomes obese as a result. The viewer cannot notice how much food s/he consumes as s/he sits and watches. Eating leads to more eating and turns the individual into a depressive one. This situation also makes the viewer asocial. Apart from TV series, video games have a similar effect on asocial personality and losing the grip on social life (Giles, 2002: 279). The diseases of the 21st century are either results or reasons for each other. As his/her brain functions slow down and s/he loses grip over life, the viewer becomes a "coach potato[2]". The viewer who loses interest in the world around stops thinking, and focusing only on the TV series, s/he becomes unable to perform even his/her daily activities. As a result, dissatisfaction appears in his family life, with kith and kin and in his/her whole social life, respectively. While the activity of watching was initially considered making use of time which would otherwise be wasted, it changes gradually, and the time which is not spent for watching would be considered wasted.

Netflix and Its Serials Used in the Research

The foundations of Netflix, a digital platform for watching TV series, was laid in Scotts Valley, California, 1997. Reed Hastings and Marc Randolph, two technology entrepreneurs, have initiated Netflix with the idea of renting DVDs online, and the concept of selling DVDs, which was a new idea at the time, attracted the audience. Since DVDs were smaller, easy to carry and with better picture quality compared to the commonly used VCDs, DVD sales started to surpass VCD sales. Moreover, the viewers were able to see the online comments regarding movies from the web page of the company and declare the type of movies they were interested in from their personal profiles. Thus, the company was able to offer movies to its customers according to their interests which was the first example of such service at the time (Wu, 2013). However, the amount of DVD players in households were still around 1 % in 1999. Receiving a boost in sales with the "five best movies to see this month" suggestions of the famous movie reviewer Leonard Maltin, Netflix offered a new application called

2 The person who spends long hours in front of the television eating junk food.

Cinematch to its followers in 2000. The application asked the users to vote at least twenty movies using stars, and the five most favorite movies selected by the interacting viewers were brought out in the Netflix web page. Netflix served its 670k members with 11500 different movies. The company's members increased to 1m in 2003, 2.6m in 2004, 4.2m in 2005, 7.5m in 2007, 20m in 2010, 27m in 2012 and 71m in 2015 (Wu, 2013).

In 2007, they added a new service apart from renting and mailing DVDs and started to stream movies online. This service, which had a motto "Watch now", was a great convenience for the viewer. Eliminating the need for waiting mails, this service became the pioneer of watching online movies. Entering the markets of Latin America and Caribbean in 2011; UK, Ireland, and Scandinavian countries in 2012 has led to a change in the shopping habits of consumers for the movie market (Wu, 2013). With its innovating online motto "watch now", Netflix started providing service in Turkey on January 6, 2016. With a free one-month trial, this service, which provides 4k resolution, can be accessed by four different devices simultaneously for a reasonable price.

The Spanish TV show *La Casa De Papel* was initially released in Antena 3 channel and finished, nevertheless, the show attracted great interest only after it was put on Netflix platform and became popular in 2018. The TV show starts telling the story of a guy nicknamed "professor" planning the greatest heist of all times and gathering collaborators. The heist is planned to be made in Royal Spanish Mint by means of printing money, and the lives of the thieves, hostages, and police officers shape with each episode. Since the show is different than the ones presenting the rich lives of the capitalist system of the 21st century, it has gained the attention of Turkish viewers in a short time by means of its different perspective.

Orange Is the New Black is an American TV show started in 2013 and has five seasons. *Orange Is the New Black* starts with an engaged woman (Piper) getting imprisoned for a couple of years because of a drug dealer she knew 10 years ago in the college. The show which mentions the struggle of the women, who has to leave her rich life with her fiancée behind and to comply with the prison conditions, is an adaptation of a novel named "My Year in a Women's Prison". Lastly, the Netflix TV show selected to be used in the study is *The Crown*, 2016. The show which has two seasons has also become popular in Turkey because of Netflix. It is a biographic TV show that follows the life of Queen Elizabeth's life and prime ministers of UK after war. The show illustrating the royal life of UK with its good and bad sides draws attention with its free manner of narrative.

Puhu TV and Its Serials Used in the Research

PuhuTV, which was founded under the roof of Doğuş Holding, is a digital platform for Turkish TV series, and started providing its services at the end of 2016. PuhuTV, which has a great number of TV series, provides its services for free unlike Netflix (PuhuTV Kullanım Koşulları, n.d.). PuhuTV shows old and current shows apart from the ones especially prepared for its digital platform, and it profits from advertisements. PuhuTV has made a name for itself especially because of the shows which cannot be followed anywhere else unless the show has finished and sold to a TV channel. The platform can be accessed by smart phones, smart TVs, and computers. Thanks to a commonly used GSM operators' support in Turkey for providing free connection while watching PuhuTV, the platform offers high resolution for its audience. PuhuTV offers a legit service and high-quality resolution options for TV shows which are hard to follow on TV channels. By means of its search engine, the platform can also identify the watching habits and taste of the users and suggest TV shows and movies accordingly and with its memory options it reminds the viewers wherever they stopped watching the show.

Its most prominent TV series is called *Fi*. Started in 2017, the show is different compared to traditional Turkish series, and it is an adaptation from the trilogy of Azra Kohen's novels; Fi, Çi and Pi. The show, whose production was undertaken by Ay Yapım, is the first PuhuTV original TV show. The show stands out with its controversial life style with its bold scenes contrary to the Turkish family's, and it narrates a famous psychologist, Can Manay who is sick himself and the frontman of a TV program falling in love with a dancer who is engaged to a man. PuhuTV became popular due to its policy to stream three episodes at once and provides a reason for binge watching.

Produced in 2018, *Şahsiyet* is another TV show especially prepared for PuhuTV just like *Fi*. The show hosts famous actors and narrates the story of a man who is under the impression that he has Alzheimer's and would forget everything in the future, thus he kills people whom he believes to be unpunished criminals; and a female police recruit trying to catch him.

Produced in 2018, *Dip* is yet another example of a crime TV series with famous actors. The show narrates the story of Sahir, a crisis negotiator, and Bilge, the daughter of a mysterious scientist. It draws further attention since the show is about the shadow government in Turkey. The show also followed the same policy of streaming three episodes at once just like *Şahsiyet* and *Fi* did, and it was suitable for binge watching.

Blutv and Its Serials Used in the Research

BluTV is owned by Doğan Group and became a digital platform in January 23, 2016 (BluTV Kurumsal İletişim Bilgileri, n.d.). BluTV has a wide variety of series: native, foreign and for children. It offers a one-month free trial and requires a reasonable subscription price afterwards. BlueTV has 30 live channels, 10k-hours-long Premium content, subtitled and dubbed alternatives, and TV shows taken from TV channels as well as the ones prepared only for BluTV; all adding to the popularity of this digital platform. BluTV, which can be watched wherever or whenever desired, is the first local online TV network in Turkey.

Masum was streamed on BluTV as the first native digital platform TV show in Turkey in January 2017. The show was presented as a miniseries, composed of eight episodes each of which lasting 60 minutes. This show was an experimental one to see the potential of Turkish digital platforms. The show had a crime drama genre, and it was about an ordinary looking Turkish family's extraordinary story. After the show ended, it was shown in Kanal D (a Turkish TV channel) yet it did not draw the same attention due to the censorship and its very late release. Therefore, *Masum* also proved the importance of digital platforms. Admiration for TV series on digital platforms, which are not shot in the TV format, reflects the desire for a free perspective.

7Yüz was another TV show on BluTV in 2017. The show had bold and uncensored scenes and narrated seven independent stories where the characters would face their darkest sides in each episode. The show was composed of 7 episodes each of which lasted 45 to 60 minutes long, and it drew interest with its unusual format as well.

Game of Thrones, which is one of the most important foreign shows of BluTV, is watched with great interest. Premiered in 2011 in USA, the fantasy genre show continued for seven seasons and got the spotlight on itself, thanks to its interesting format and high budged. BluTV by means of adding one of the most popular American production TV show to its digital platform has enabled its followers to simultaneously watch the episodes with the USA audience. The show has managed to take people's minds from the real world by means of its unusual format, shocking deaths of the characters, and its fantastic world.

Dizimag5.Co and Its Serials Used in the Research

The reason for the selection of Dizimag5.co is because the foreign shows fit for binge watching are usually streamed in alternative digital TV show platforms. TV series such as *Supernatural* and *Grey's Anatomy* are most popular American shows whose seasons the viewers would like to binge watch. Unlike Turkish shows, their episodes are 45 minutes long.

Supernatural started in September 13, 2005 and completed its 13th season in 2018. The American show has been rewarded with 28 awards including 1 Golden Globe and 6 Emmys. The show narrates the story of two unyielding brothers who try to save the world by means of hunting supernatural creatures. The concepts of god, angels, and devil take inspiration from John Milton's epic poem "Paradise Lost" (Milton and Martin, 1846). "Paradise Lost" is a 350-year old poem written by John Milton who was blind; however, he described paradise and hell as if he was there and reinterpreted the exile of humans from paradise. The show uses the poem's content for the depiction of angels and demons and even for their names, and the show brings a different perspective to Christianity with its religious references. The show is watched with great appreciation around the world.

Grey's Anatomy is an American show which was adapted into a Turkish version called *Doktorlar* when the original show was at its 13th season. The American show started in March 27, 2005 and completed its 14th season in 2018. The show narrating the story of doctors specializing in their fields, their experiences, and the lives of patients visiting the hospital is still very popular in USA and many other countries. It has been awarded with various Emmys and Golden Globes, and it is ideal for Binge Watching.

The Research and Its Results

This study examines the following via focus group discussion: what affects the choices of the viewers on digital streaming platforms such as *Netflix, PuhuTV, BluTV, dizimag5.co* while selecting a show to watch; whether these viewers have a habit of binge watching, and if so, how binge watching affects them emotionally. Twenty people aging between 19 and 29 years or 30 and 39 years and including students and academicians from various departments (Radio Television and Cinema, English Language and Literature, Public Relations, Translation and Interpreting -English, Russian and Arabic-, English Language Teaching, New Media English, Audiology and Dentistry) of both state and private universities in Turkey (Istanbul University, Marmara University, Beykent University, Gelisim University, Istanbul Aydin University and Istanbul Bilgi University) were chosen as the focus group. The only condition in the selection of the group of 10 men and 10 women was having watched all of the seasons of the shows (*La Casa De Papel, Orange is the New Black, The Crown, Fi, Şahsiyet, Dip, Supernatural, Grey's Anatomy, Masum, 7Yüz* ve *Game of Thrones*) included in the study.

The questions asked during the discussions are based on binge watching. Moreover, the participants were asked the reason for selecting these 11 shows and if they identify themselves with the characters while watching.

1. Do you have a subscription to any of the following streaming services: PuhuTV, Netfix, BluTV ve dizimag5.co? If so, why? If you have two or more subscription which do you prefer the most? Why?
2. Which of the following shows do you feel close to or watch the most: *La Casa De Papel* (2017), *Orange is the New Black* (2013), *The Crown* (2016), *Fi* (2017), *Sahsiyet* (2018), *Dip* (2018), *Supernatural* (2005) ve *Grey's Anatomy* (2005), *Masum* (2017), *7Yuz* (2017) ve *Game of Thrones* (2011)?
3. Have you ever identified yourself with one or some of the characters from *La Casa De Papel* (2017), *Orange is the New Black* (2013), *The Crown* (2016), *Fi* (2017), *Sahsiyet* (2018), *Dip* (2018), *Supernatural* (2005) ve *Grey's Anatomy* (2005), *Masum* (2017), *7Yuz* (2017) ve *Game of Thrones* (2011)? If you have, which character and why?
4. Which of the following shows do you think is the most nerve-shredding? Why? Have you ever watched any of the shows in rapid succession without even leaving your seat? If so, how many episodes did you watch at one go and for how long?
5. Have you ever neglected or forgotten something important or performing daily tasks that you had to do just because you were too caught up in watching? If so, how did you feel once you realized that you had forgotten?
6. What do you feel while watching a TV show? Do you watch it on your free time or do you actually make time for that?
7. Have you ever felt any physical discomfort? If so, how did you feel? Did you see a doctor?
8. Are you able to think about something else while watching a TV show? Or is it watching a show or a movie that keeps your mind off thinking about other things?

The focus group study took 120 minutes. The interviews were recorded, and each participant was informed that the data would be used in a binge watching study and deciphered. Popular TV shows, which are ideal for binge watching, were selected for the research.

For the first question, all the participants answered that they had a PuhuTV membership and they preferred this platform because it was free. The participants confessed that while this habit was for spending their free time at first, it changed into one they started to create time for when they discovered they could watch TV shows without any time or location restriction. The participants also mentioned that they only did not want to watch dizimag5.co TV shows anywhere else other than their computers, and that they desired Turkish platforms of foreign shows to include more TV shows without any delay compared to their American counterparts.

3 out of 5 female participants aging 19–29 and 2 out of 5 female participants from the 30–39 group stated that they had a Netflix subscription. Rest of the female participants (5) stated that they were following Netflix shows from alternative sources, but their desire to watch these shows was due to Netflix. BluTV has the smallest number of female subscribers out of 10 participants. It is stated that the TV shows of BluTV were watched by 4 of the female participants when it was released on TV, another 4 watched them during the free trial, and the last 2 continued their subscription after the trial was over. It was found out that, from the 19–29 group, 3 of the male participants had Netflix subscription, and 2 participants had the free trial of BluTV. The 30–39 group, on the other hand, has 4 participants with Netflix subscription, and 2 of them has both Netflix and BluTV subscription.

3 out of 5 female participants from the 19–29 group mentioned that they found *Game of Thrones* interesting because the show had a fantasy world which they enjoyed when they were bored with their monotonous lives. They stated that they felt themselves closer to the character Khaleesi Daenery Targaryen because she presented a strong female character and she was more honest and braver compared to many male kings. They even mentioned that Turkish women are also fighters just like the Khaleesi. Another female participant stated that despite following foreign TV shows, she favored the Turkish show *Sahsiyet* as well and she identified herself with the female police officer of the show. When she was asked why she identified herself with this character, she mentioned that despite the character is considered weak, she has subtle wit and a female perspective to solve the problems where other males fail, thus she proves how patient and resilient she is and helps raising consciousness that Turkish women are needed in every field. Another participant mentioned that she favored the show *La Casa de Papel* because of the plentiful action and felt herself close to the character called Tokyo. She explained her liking for Tokyo that this powerful and brave female character reminded her that there is always a way out in life even in the most hopeless moments.

Two female participants from the 30–39 group have answered the 2nd and 3rd questions stating that they felt closer to *Grey's Anatomy*. The reason for their choice was because they wanted to live in the free world Meredith Grey has, and they considered themselves as successful and persistent as her. The other 3 female participants stated that they liked Turkish shows more, and despite that they cannot fully identify themselves with any of the characters in the show, their favorite shows is *Fi*. They further added they might prefer the combination of 2 female characters from this show which resembles foreign shows. They stated that the two main characters, Duru and Ozge, had similar features like themselves; strong, stubborn, and aware of their desires.

3 of the male participants from the 19–29 group said that they liked *Game of Thrones* and the character Jon because of his steadfast attitude. The other 2 in the group mentioned that they liked the Professor in La Casa de Papel because, they themselves had similar characteristics of being a cunning and silent person nobody can understand. 3 of the male participants from the 30–39 group also preferred *Game of Thrones* and the character Jon. Another from the middle age group identified himself with the character Berlin from *La Casa de Papel* because, he had control over his life with his rules just like this character. The last participant from this group stated that he liked the character Sahir from *Dip* because this character was helping suicidal people in a heroic manner, and the participant's job was made him feel the same way when he is helping people.

The answers of 4th, 5th and 6th questions showed that majority of the 19–29 group thought all the 11 TV shows were escapist as if their episodes were designed to be watched all at once. The participants stated that they are interested in TV series, and they watched the series in the research because of their popularity. Participants also mentioned that they usually lost the track of time while watching and even did not leave home for 2 to 3 days, and they would like to have a similar experience of watching in the future if they could find an escapist show. The longest time of watching without break was 36 hours on 2 seasons for 2 female participants, and 32 hours on 2 seasons for 2 male participants. The shortest time of watching, including the time for necessary breaks, was 3 hours a day. The participants suggested that the minimum number of episodes to be watched at once was 2 episodes, and they supported the policy of Turkish digital platforms to present 3 episodes together which enabled them to have a movie-like experience.

Both male and female participants of the 30–39 group also thought that these 11 TV shows were escapist, but they could not always find the free time to watch them because of their jobs and families; thus, they especially spared time for the watching activity at the weekends losing track of time and even ignoring their daily tasks. They have also commented that the very aim of the TV series was giving an escape to them from their responsibilities and an opportunity of isolation from their troubles; therefore, they even spent their lunch break on digital platforms. This group's minimum and maximum watching time is 1 hour and 5 hours, respectively.

Tab. 1: Show and Character Preferences of the Participants

The Show	Those who prefer the show	Character preference	Reason for Preference of the Character
Game of Thrones	3 Females (Aged 19–29)	Khaleesi	Role model as a strong woman, more honest and braver than the kings and being a warrior
	3 Males (Aged 19–29)	Jon Snow	His strong look and personal trait as one never giving up
	3 Males (Aged 30–39)	Jon Snow	His strong look and personal trait as one never giving up
La Casa De Papel	1 Female (Aged 19–29)	Tokio	That she reminds us there can be a way out even in the most desperate moments of life, and her being a strong and brave woman.
	2 Males (Aged 19–29)	The Professor	Their personal traits such as being clever, crafty, and quiet just like the Professor
	1 Males (Aged 30–39)	Berlin	That they feel as if they dominated the world with their own rules just like Berlin
Fi	3 Females (Aged 30–39)	Duru and Ozge	That they discover themselves through such personal traits of Duru and Ozge as being strong, stubborn, and knowing what they want
Grey's Anatomy	2 Females (Aged 30–39)	Meredith Grey	Wanting live in a free world as Meredith Grey has and seeing themselves as fighters and successful
Sahsiyet	1 Female (Aged 19–29)	Female Police Officer	Her solving crimes subtly and in a better way than the male police officers, making her difference felt by the others and proving she is durable and patient
Dip	1 Males (Aged 30–39)	Sahir	Feeling that they are also a hero at work and helping others like Sahir who helps those who are suicidal

Tab. 2: Duration of Nonstop Watching by Age

Age Group	Maximum Duration of Watching	Minimum Duration of Watching
Ages 19–29	2 seasons in 32–36 hours	3 hours
Ages 30–39	5 hours	1 hour

According to the answers of 7th and 8th questions, the participants of 19–29 group felt a sensation of numbness and tingling on their arms and legs but they did not feel the need to consult a physician in such times; instead they gave a break to recover from this state. Only 1 of the male participants mentioned that he had no discomfort.

The male and female participants of the 30–39 group also reported swelling and tingling on their arms and legs. 2 of the female participants consulted a physician with such complaints, and they were told the problem was caused by lack of activity-related edema, and they were advised to engage in physical activities. 2 male and 3 female participants confessed that they gained a lot of weight while watching and almost became obese; however, they could not help themselves watching TV series.

It was stated that the participants did not only stop thinking while watching; they did not want to think at all, and they were all of one mind about the reason of watching that it is for emptying their minds. 3 females and 2 males from the 30–39 group and 2 females and 1 male from the 19–29 group have claimed that the watching activity became more than just spending their free time; they started to spare time for watching and did not consider getting involved in other activities before finishing the seasons of a specific TV show they are engaged in.

Young and middle-aged participants of the focus group study have overall stated that they became addicted to TV series. It is found out that the majority of female participants identified themselves with strong female characters and took examples of them. Similarly, the male participants identified themselves with strong, intelligent, and libertarian characters.

It was found out in the study that both male and female characters went beyond spending their free time and created time for the activity of watching; they also suffered physical discomfort during the process, and some of them consulted a physician due to such problems. The participants who spent at least an hour for a 60 minutes long episode confessed that they even forgot performing their daily tasks while watching TV shows. It was also observed that the participants who watched at least 3 episodes of 45 minutes long foreign TV shows identified the problem of addiction, although they were unfamiliar with the term “binge watching”.

Conclusion

Digital media shows have become a popular tool of consumption, thanks to their various features; easy access from different devices and different locations, uncensored content, and a great range of options. This USA-pioneered market, due to the great number of addicting shows, has brought a new digital habit called "binge watching". According to the results of a study conducted in USA, 2013, 67 % of the viewers, aged 13 to 39, watched a season without break (MarketCast, 2013). It was proved in a study made on TiVo[3] in 2014 that 91 % of the viewers had a habit of binge watching (Marketwatch, 2014). This study with its focus groups also serves a proof that this habit is becoming widespread in Turkey at a similar rate.

It has been observed in the study that the viewers who experienced binge watching once would like to repeat this experience. As the study focuses men and women separately, it was found out that women have the habit of watching 5.4 % higher than men which is not a significant difference. Therefore, it has been concluded that the habit of watching TV series is critically high both for women and for men in Turkey. It was also claimed by the participants that their habits were partly because of the great variety of TV series and movies online; one can watch a movie from the 1960s or a recently released one in 2018 which makes him/her feel free. Participants also mentioned that their preference for the digital platforms was also because they could be accessed through mobile applications. Furthermore, they mentioned that online public comments from the digital platforms gave them some ideas about the shows and had an influence over their choices. It was found out that the watching habits of viewers aged 19 to 39 have changed; the viewers stated that digital platforms are more attractive due to their features like nonrestriction of time and location, uncensored content, ability to access from different devices which enables them watch without interruption.

Another point which was questioned in the study was if the viewers preferred the series in which they felt a bond with the characters. One way or another, all the participants have expressed that they identified themselves with the characters in TV series and this became a determinant in the way they felt closer to the show. The biggest gender difference, in terms of the characters the viewers find themselves closer to even though their favorite show stays the same, is seen in *Game of Thrones*. In the focus group of 20, 9 picked the shows as their favorite and women identified themselves with Khaleesi while men do with Jon Snow. However, the reason for choosing the show stays the same: that they find these characters strong and brave.

Participants were asked about the duration of their long and continuous watching. In the 19–29 age group, 2 female participants reported that they watched 2 seasons in 36 hours and 2 male participants in 2 seasons in 32 hours.

The shortest non-stop watching time among participants is 3 hours per day. In the 30–39 age group, these periods fall: not more than 5 hours, at least 1 hour. Participants, who stated that they did not want to think about something, not that they could not think of, while watching the series, generally agree that the purpose of watching the series is to empty their minds. 8 of the 20 participants emphasized that the habit of watching a series is no longer a leisure time activity, but they actually make time to watch the series.

It was also pointed out by the participants that binge watching could lead to some physical and psychological disorders. Participants mentioned having a sensation of numbness and tingling on their legs when watching TV series for a long duration. Moreover, the study indicates that this habit could lead to obesity, and the individuals with lack of activity might face serious heart and blood pressure problems in the long term. The precise effects of excessive eating, watching and sitting in the long term will be determined with another research in the future. Considering the increasing number of digital platforms and the online habits of young generation in particular, It is determined that the market of TV series will keep growing in the digital platforms, and the number of disorders such as binge watching will increase.

With their rapidly increasing number of users/viewers and their disruptive structure on the boundaries of real and dream world, digital platforms are a threat to the young and middle-aged population and require precautions to be taken. Despite the fact that digital platforms are necessary, it must be explained to the viewer that TV series, movies, video games and other programs should be accessed with limitation. To raise consciousness of the public, the physical and psychological side effects should be explained by means of public service announcements. These platforms, which are initially used to spend free time, have the adverse effect of creating free time for watching TV series and playing games, and consequently, moving youth away from the reality and causing them to put off life.

Bibliography

Baudrillard, J. (2010). Tüketim Toplumu: Söylenceleri/Yapıları. (H. Deliceçaylı & F. Keskin, Trans.). İstanbul: Ayrıntı Yayınları.

Bentham, J. (1995). The Panopticon Writings. New York: Verso.

BluTV Kurumsal İletişim Bilgileri. (n.d.). Retrieved from https://destek.blutv.com.tr/hc/tr/articles/115001677605-BluTV-Kurumsal-%C4%B0leti%C5%9Fim-Bilgileri on 25 May 2018.

Fontaine, G. (2013). Television 2025: Video as a Service. Communications & Strategies, Fourth Quarter, 2013(92), 115–123.

Gay, V. (2013, July 3). How will Binge Watching Change TV? Newsday.com. Retrieved from http://www.newsday.com/entertainment/tv/how-willbinge-watching-change-tv-1.5619328 on 12 December 2018.

Gerbner, G. (2002). On Content Analysis and Critical Research in Mass Communication. In M. Morgan (Ed.), Against the Mainstream (pp. 75–82). New York: Peter Lang.

Giles, D. C. (2002). Parasocial Interaction: A Review of the Literature and a Model for Future Research. Media Psychology, 4(3), 279–305.

Huxley, A. (2007). Brave New World. Toronto: Vintage.

Jurgensen, J. (2012, July 13). Binge Viewing: TV's Lost Weekends. WSJ.com. Retrieved from http://online.wsj.com/news/articles/SB100014240527023037 407045775213008 06686174.25-32 on 23 November 2018.

Kristeva, J. (2017). Ruhun Yeni Hastalıkları (N. Tutal, Trans.). İstanbul: Ayrıntı Yayınları.

Marketcast. (2013). Market Cast Study Finds TV "Binge-Watching" Creates a More Engaged Viewer for Future Seasons and Not a Bingeing Habit. Retrieved from http://www.prewb.com/releases/2013/3/prewb10513066.htm on 3 February 2019.

Marketwatch. (2014). Viewers' New TV Reality: "A Season"=One Day. Retrieved from http://www.marketwatch.com/story/viewers-new-tv-reality-a season-one-day-2014-06-25 on 19 December 2018.

Milton, J. & Martin, J. (1846). The Paradise lost of John Milton. London: Charles Whittingham.

Netflix Kurumsal Bilgileri. (n.d.). Retrieved from https://help.netflix.com/tr/node/2101 on 14 September 2018.

Orwell, G. (2008). Nineteen Eighty-Four. London: Penguin Books.

Oxford Dictionaries. (2013). Word of the Year 2013: Runners-up. Retrieved from http:/blog.oxforddictionaries.com/2013/11/Word-of-the-year-runners-up/ on 4 October 2018.

Postman, N. (2014). Televizyon: Öldüren Eğlence Gösteri Çağında Kamusal Söylem (O. Akınhay, Trans.). İstanbul: Ayrıntı Yayınları.

PuhuTV Kullanım Koşulları. (n.d.). Retrieved from https://puhutv.com/kullanim-kosullari on 12 September 2018.

Ramsay. (2013, October 4). Confessions of a Binge Watcher. Retrieved from https://cstonline.net/confessions-of-a-binge-watcher-by-debra-ramsay/. on 29 October 2018.

Wu, T. (2013, December 4). Netflix's War on Mass Culture. NewRepublic.com. Retrieved from http://www.newrepublic.com/article/115687/netflixswar-mass-culture. on 23 October 2018.

Yengin, D. & Kınay, Ö. (2015). Yeni Medyada Boş Zamanın Dönüşümü: Tıkınmalı İzleme. In D. Yengin (Ed.), Sosyal Medya Araştırmaları (pp. 213–257). İstanbul: Paloma Yayınları.

Özge Topçu

Online Narcissism

Abstract: This chapter tackles ego surfing. As known, one of the terms that have become popular together with the proliferation of the internet use is the internet surfing. However, now that what is being searched on the internet has become the individual himself or herself, another problem called ego surfing comes into existence. Ego surfing is described as the behavior in which some of the people who are fond of technology constantly search for their own names on the internet and follow the updates regarding their lives, feel happy when they find any information or like for them, but discomfort otherwise. The study concentrates on the definition of online narcissism, how it has emerged, and how it can be dealt with. A survey with 20 questions, it has been aimed to determine the users' internet addiction, their perception for the extent to which they are narcissist, and how often they search for their names.

Keywords: narcissism, online narcissism, ego-surfing, technology addiction, digital disorder, generation Z

Introduction

Technology has developed greatly, and it has become inevitable in people's lives in today's world. Whereas technology makes people's lives easier, the selves remain under the captivity of technology. Thanks to smartphones, people can access the internet at any time in many places and they become more committed to the screen. However, the overuse of internet causes quite serious problems. The people, putting the internet in the heart of their lives, might be on the verge of detaching themselves from social life. Furthermore, some of them who are addicted to the internet quite care about the comments, criticisms, or admiration given for themselves, and they spend most of the time on following these things. Today, when people are just a click away from everything, the technology causes some disorders and behavioral disorders to occur. One of them is "ego-surfing" that is defined as some of the people who are addicted to the internet search for their names on the internet periodically and follow the news about themselves (Gündüz, 2007). Another term of ego-surfing disorder is online narcissism. The people, who have a narcissistic personality disorder, have an inflated sense of their own importance and they always look for admiration and interest (Atkinson et al. 1995: 643). This study focuses on the definition of "online narcissism", how it has occurred, and how it can be treated.

The present age is called internet age. The understanding that internet addiction and collateral disorders should be regarded as disorders or behavioral disorders needing treatment in the process occurs. Carrying the life without internet is getting harder. Leading a life without internet is getting harder. Addiction is described as a recurrent and chronic brain disorder regardless of its harmful consequences (Başkurt, 2003: 75). Besides this, addictions such as gambling, shopping, sports, drinking, and smoking, that the technology also causes addiction in the brain, is stated on the researches made (Tarhan and Nurmedov, 2013: 21). That the computer and the internet take place under the category of addiction is seen. According to Tarhan (2013: 9), the computer and internet are useful tools in terms of communication and knowledge acquisition, however, that the users use the technology mostly for communication due to the increase in communication is seen after the improvement in the field of technology. The technology addiction takes the place of friendship of technology. The internet is an important tool with regards to enabling people to reach the information demanded and communicate with each other. Whereas the problems, which people have, are raised because of technology usage, they spend much more time on the internet to cope up with these problems (Dinç, 2010: 42). Those people, overusing the internet, are sensitive to the disappointment they had in their relationships is observed.

People's social relations are developed with regards to other people's behaviors and skills on the internet or games. At this point, that habits have an important role and internet environments cause identity to be changed is observed. The internet is more encouraging than television. People, addicted to the internet, want to refrain from reality under stress and, head to the internet. Tarhan states that these people are more alone and feel depressed than nonaddicted people (Tarhan, 2013: 72). The disorders and behavioral disorders show up in different ways according to how people use the internet and their habits.

Digital disorders show up in different ways. Whereas that people consistently search for the people around themselves on the internet is defined as "Google follow-up", that people search for their names on the internet is defined as "ego-surfing" (Duygulu, 2017). That they follow likes, comments, and sharing about themselves closely is an obvious symptom of ego-surfing ("Teknoloji 'e-hastalıkları' doğurdu", 2017). Nowadays, social webs are popular communication tools. The act that *"People share their feelings and ideas"* expressed in the definition of communication is carried out on social media (Güngör, 2011: 111). The psychological disorders related to the overuse of social media are increased as a result of developments in digital technology and the spread of social media. *"Smartphone fasting"* is said to be one of the ways to cope up with the digital disorders. The specialists state that if people do not use electronic devices, that situation would cause a kind of "digital detox", so they could get rest (Schumann & Topçu, 2013). We should pay more attention to the topic of technology addiction in children and youngsters.

New technologies make people's lives easier and raise their living standards; however, new problems occur (Andreassen vd., 2012: 85; Çam and İşbulan, 2012; 51). The internet is one of the inevitable things in our lives. Accessing the internet, both fast and cheap, causes an increase in its uses rapidly. The time spent on the internet brings out different effects. Furthermore, it is also possible to encounter with so many physical and mental problems. One of these problems, internet addiction, can be seen in every age and sex.

The internet is regarded as an application causing addiction. However, social media addiction, digital media addiction, and smartphone addiction are more specific issues and their focus is the addiction. The time spent on mass-communication tools is decreased due to the internet. The internet also affects face-to-face social relations. People have begun to prefer spending time on the internet, social media, or other innovations to having a chat in a place. After the developments in the internet technology, people are addicted to the internet due to more common use of smartphones and tablets. If the technology addiction is not treated, the situation might get worse. This study, together with its survey questions, aims to specify how much people use the internet, find out their addiction levels, and how much they are active on ego-surfing.

Technology Addiction

Each new technology has pros and cons. One of the cons is technology and internet addiction. The overuse of technology damages both people's daily lives and their relations. Nevzat Tarhan states that young people "ego-surf" on the internet, satisfy their egos, and spend both too much energy and time due to their internet addiction (T.C. Üsküdar Üniversitesi, 2017). He expresses that the new generation is the social media generation, and it is more difficult to lead the new generation than other generations. Besides, according to Tarhan (Tarhan, 2017), this generation rejects to some issues; however, they accept their current situation and circumstances, and Tarhan evaluates this situation in a positive way.

Addiction is one of the biggest problems of our age. However, when we say addiction, chemical addictions come to mind first, and they are categorized as heroin, alcohol, and smoking addiction. Nevertheless, the issue of addiction is more than that, it has much broader meaning. Addiction is a syndrome. Addiction is scrutinized under two categories such as behavioral and physical addictions. When we analyze the differences between physical and psychological addictions, it is possible to state that people might be addicted to both at the same time; however, it is easier to treat physical addiction than psychological addiction. The reason is that getting rid of psychological addiction depends on them and this process requires a long therapy (Öztürk et al., 2007: 15). There are some criteria such as emotional changes, deprivation, tolerance, and interpersonal conflict that a behavior should have been counted as an addiction.

The term "addiction" is defined as *"addiction to a physical item"*. Addiction is a situation that disturbs people mentally and emotionally in their daily lives. In that period, they might have difficulty in observing their own situations; thus, it is important for others around them to follow their situation closely (Düvenci, 2012: 87). A new term "internet addiction" has been recently added to the terms coined related to addiction. Internet addiction, appearing with the indications such as people spending too much time on the internet, not being able to control themselves on the issue of time spent on the internet, and beginning to panic when the internet is not available, is an interesting topic having been discussed in psychiatry literature from the 1990s until today (Özsoy, 2009: 651). The term "internet addiction" was coined by Goldberg in 1996. Goldberg, making the definition of "inappropriate internet use causing a clinical disorder", build indicators for internet addiction in accordance with diagnostic criteria for drug abuse (as cited in Suler, 1996). Also, Young carries similar studies and specified 8 indicators for internet addiction. Young asserts that if a person has 5 out of these indicators, he can be diagnosed as "addicted to the internet". These indicators are as follows: 1) surfing on the internet very much, 2) needing to use internet excessively to have fun, 3) inadequate attempts with regards to decreasing the time spent on the internet, 4) anxiety felt in case the time used on the internet decreases, 5) spending time on the internet more than planned, 6) having problems with people from his school, family, and work due to overuse of internet, 7) lying to others about the time spent on the internet, 8) using the internet especially for getting away from the problems (Bozkurt et al. 2016: 15). The group, especially between 12 and 18, bears the risk of being addicted to the internet, and this situation is possible to be seen in every age group. The addiction rate of young people in their adolescence period is quite high as they regard their phones as a part of their personalities (Hooper and Zhou, 2007: 101).

That 23.2 percent of the students are addicted to the internet and 28.4 percent are internet users at risk is seen in the study done among students at Selçuk University. 51.6 percent of attendants are problematic internet users. According to this study, internet users are at risk and the addicted ones spend time on the internet every day or 4–5 days every week (Balcı and Gülnar: 2009: 6). People, addicted to the internet, spend more time on social media and spend less time with their friends. These people do not spend time with their families as much as they do on social media (Kim et al. 2008: 214). On one hand, people satisfy some needs via social media; on the other hand, they might encounter with some danger. The problems such as addiction, sleep disorders, and some physical pain occur because of overuse of social media (Andreassen et al., 2012: 85; Çam and İşbulan: 2012: 25). One of the distinctive factors of social media use, narcissism, is a remarkable factor. People, having narcissistic character features, usually share more photos and write more (Ong et al., 2011: 57).

The internet has become an inevitable part of people's daily lives. However, the overuse of internet, for other purposes than searching for information on the internet and making social interaction easier, causes an increase in internet addiction. One of the features of digital media is that sharing is possible with an appropriate protocol, the interface is connected to the other, and people on different geographical areas can share among each other easily, thanks to the network (Feldman, 1997:15). McLuhan states that technological improvements structure the communication and the tool affects the content of communication. Thus, when the tool is changed, the communication type is changed. Therefore, it is possible to say that technological improvements and the change of tools affect the communication type. According to Roger, the new media is different from other medias with these three features: demassification, interactivity, asynchronousity (as cited in Geray, 2003:18).

Digital media refers to the contents such as digitally compressed sound and video photographs. There are a lot of data on the internet as the contents are on digital media (Kelleci, 2008: 254). All kind of information is transferred to the people and the society on the media. Moreover, digital media is effective in molding public opinion and manipulate the people. Thanks to the improvements in communication technologies, the handicaps related to time and place on digital media tools are removed. Digital media tools have become cheaper in time and it is easy to access them. Thus, digital media is important in every sphere of life and an inevitable part of people's daily lives. This situation has caused human affairs to be replaced by the relations between the screen and the person, and make people become addicted to digital media tools. So many problems such as an increase in musculoskeletal disorders due to digital media addiction and eye dryness and sleep disorders occur due to standing still and looking at the screen for so long time (Ulukol, 2013: 120).

The narcissistic people can thrust themselves forward on social networks as social webs give an opportunity for people to demonstrate themselves as how they associate themselves with their inner self (Buffardi and Campbell, 2008: 15).

People present themselves as how they want via social media. If a person is shy about communicating face-to-face with other people in their daily lives, he demonstrates himself as a quite active person on social media. This situation makes the person's psychology change on social media. Social media addiction is a problem and the overuse causes people to have problems such as low academic performance, sleep disorders, and relationship problems. The internet is significant in students' school lives; thus, the time of using the internet increases due to things the internet supplies. This situation also increases the possibility of students to be at risk.

The internet addiction is a topic drawing the ever-increasing attention of the researches recently. The overuse of internet for some people is an addiction and that is regarded as a reason for anxiety (Griffiths, 1998: 73). The internet addiction is "being addicted to the internet psychologically apart from things being done on the internet after connected to the internet". People addicted to the internet use the internet to get away from the problems in their lives rather than searching for information on the internet (Kandell,1998: 12). People become addicted to the internet as they let themselves be affected by the influence of device just like alcohol addiction. Internet addiction is different from the chemical addictions in terms of it affecting the behaviors (Thurlow et al., 2004: 159).

Especially, the importance of misusing and addiction for the behavioral addictions makes the definition of addictions difficult. Vaillant states that *"we should liken the addiction to a mountain or a season and see it like something which you could feel when you experience instead of finding a definition for it"* (as cited in Kurtaran, 2008: 8). Although it was firstly defined as internet addiction, the researches begin to define it in a different way in time. These are internet dependency, pathological internet use, problematic internet use, excessive internet use, internet abuse, and internet addiction disorder. Young and Goldberg, making researches about internet addiction, have preferred the term *"internet addiction"* (Dinç, 2010: 17).

That there is no restriction for the time spent on the internet, they can always benefit from the internet, they can share their real ideas without feeling shy, they can easily communicate with people all around the world, people having same tastes can meet, they can communicate with others spending minimum time and money, they have the right to cease communicating whenever they want, they can introduce themselves as they wish, they can economically access entertainment and games, they feel equal to others, and they have a lot of choices to escape from daily tension are some attractive features of internet (Dinç, 2010: 40). The technology, useful for people in terms of communicating or sharing information, might be dangerous if they do not use it properly. The people addicted to the internet are people, who are happy when connected to the internet, wanting to prolong the time as far as possible on the internet and resisting in case they are restrained. One of the reasons under this behavior is the appeal of virtual world.

Narcissism in the Context of Personality and Ego

The notion of idiosyncratic personality is acquired with the combination of innate characters' traits and environmental factors. People, who can satisfy their needs with the society without having any problems, are healthy. An ordinary human being identifies his desires and requests with society's expectation. One of the approaches related to becoming a society is ego/self-formation. Having a happy life first depends on the person and then on the environment. The person should have a healthy personality development for this. Ego enables people to understand the reality, comply with it, think and find solutions to the obstacles faced (Yurdagül, 1987: 1). W. James, having developed the theory of ego, divides the ego under two groups such as "known me" and "knowing I". The ego is a source explaining the questions about how the behaviors occur. The term "ego" is particularly based on the ideas of George Herbert, Mead and Charles Horton Cooley in the sociology (Coştu, 2009: 126). The personality and ego-formation in the sociology are possible in a specific society (Kurtkan, 1979: 24). The personality is an acquired feature distinguishing the person from the others. The personality comes out at the end of the continuity of a person's mental, social, and emotional features. At this point, it is possible to say that personality is an important factor designating the behavior and relationship forms.

Narcissism is defined as an inflated ego term (Campbell et al., 2002: 361). The narcissistic people act according to their own benefits. Although they do not have a satisfactory success in a subject area, they think exactly the opposite. They would like to be recognized as distinguished people. They usually behave selfishly in interpersonal communication. They enjoy revealing the weak points of others and use against them. They do not care about what others think. They are jealous people in general. However, they extremely like themselves. The term "narcissistic personality disorder" is defined as *"superiority-ego and the will to be liked by others"* (Köroğlu and Bayraktar, 2007: 25). Particularly Kohut carried out remarkable studies related to narcissisim. According to Kohut, narcissism is a part of the normal development process. Narcissistic people are defined as people whose needs were not met in their childhood by their parents and thus, they try to fulfill their needs, not being met, in their adulthood.

Phenomenon of Online Narcissism

Whereas smoking, alcohol, and drug are considered as addictions in society, we can say that technology and the internet are serious kinds of addiction. People spend so much time on the internet that they might get away from life after a while and they could remain insensitive to the world. Reaching the information easily makes life easier. And people spending most of their time with the technology and feeling angry if they cannot access are regarded as addicted.

Some of technophile people search for their names on the internet periodically and follow the events about their posts, likes, comments, or reports. Some of these people might have been caught the "ego-surfing" disorder, one of the behavioral disorders. Another term of ego-surfing is "online narcissism". Narcissism is defined as *"liking yourself"*. Ego-surfing is the reflection of people's liking themselves in the social world. These people follow the likes, sharing, and comments closely and search for these on the internet. Phones are not used just for communication anymore. They are used to check e-mails and to take videos and photos. Furthermore, they are useful in so many areas about the job and become an important part of people' lives. Whereas they are so important in people' lives, mobile phones make people addicted in time (Polat, 2017: 5). Although the term "ego-surfing", defined as *"searching for people's their own names on the internet periodically and look for information about themselves"*, was added to the Oxford English Dictionary in 1998, it goes back to the time when internet showed up. The aims of people ego-surfing are different. Whereas some people search on the internet to satisfy their ego, others dream of millions reading information about themselves.

Narcissistic people might get angry if others do not respond to their sharing. It is possible to say that these people always anticipate others admiring them and they think that they are more precious and important in their relations. Besides, these individuals are highly greedy when it comes to verbalizing the interests and admires directed to themselves while they act without caring about others' situations. The digital addiction is a topic, which should be taken seriously. The only thing that matters is being able to control themselves. Some ways to get rid of the addiction are such as: utilizing the positive sides of technology, being aware of that and receiving psychological support when they feel desperate.

Method

With the development of technology, it is seen that that the number of people having digital disorders, behavioral disorder, and pathological use have increased every day. People are aware of these disorders or not. The aims of this study are to reveal what the users know about ego-surfing and how it effects on the users. In this research, it has been researched that what online narcissism is and what its effects are on the users through randomized sampling technique.

The universe of the research consists of the Generations X, Y, and Z. Whereas the Generations X and Y spend some time on the internet, the Generation Z cannot imagine a life without internet. We look for which generations search for their names on the internet in the study, and we expect that particularly the Generations Y and Z would be determinant. The information about which method is followed is provided in the method part of the research. The steps such as explaining the problem and how it can be solved are included in the research (Aziz, 2015: 31).

As the technique of data collection, the survey technique in the quantitative category is applied. In the quantitative method, a planned, representative sample and statistic procedure should be carried out (Yengin, 2017: 60). The reason for choosing this method is to measure the effects of ego-surfing, one of the digital disorders, on the users, specify how well the users know it and evaluate this according to the data acquired from survey result. The data such as questions and comments related to online narcissism are gathered in the survey study consisting of twenty questions. 382 people participated in the survey. The survey starts with measuring demographic information and continues with asking questions to the participants about internet use. Then, the participants' opinions and comments regarding ego-surfing are asked.

The survey is carried out with the primary school, secondary school, and high school graduates and people having bachelor's, master's, and doctorate degrees between the dates of 18.04.2018 and 15.05.2018. The questions related to the rate of people having online narcissism, its effect on people, and its connection with narcissism take place in the last part of survey, consisting of twenty questions. For example, most of the people giving the answer "I agree" to the question such as "ego-surfing is a sign of narcissism" indicate that how effective the connection between the ego-surfing and narcissism is, and people ego-surfing have narcissistic features. As high school graduates' rate is high with 40 %, it is possible to state that this group is determinant on the survey result. Whereas 52 % of participants spend between 2 and 4 hours on the internet, people spending between 0 and 1 hour represent 4 % of all with the lowest rate. This fact shows that people spend at least 2 hours on the internet. People expressing that they use their mobile phones at a high rate, such as 80 %, when spending time on the internet indicates that their mobile phones are in the heart of people's lives.

Tab. 1: Demographics of Participants

Groups	**Frequency**	**Percentage (%)**
Sex		
Female	146	61
Male	236	39
Age		
13–18	132	37
19–24	47	12
25–30	28	8
31–36	62	16
37 and over	113	27
Education		
Primary School	22	4
Secondary School	4	1
High School	143	40
Bachelor	153	38
Master	58	15
Doctorate	2	2

Findings

382 people attended the online survey. The demographic information about attendants, the time they spent on the internet, the devices they used to connect to the internet, the information they have about ego-surging, the relation between digital disorders and narcissism, and rate of catching to ego-surfing disorder are calculated on the survey.

When the demographic data of survey is analyzed, that 61 % are women and 39 % are men is seen. That women attended the survey more or they are more liable to answer the survey questions is seen. When we look at the age range of attendants, it has been observed that people between 13 and 18 attended at most with a rate of 37 %. As people born after 2000 are accepted as the Generation Z, it is understood that the survey was responded by mostly the Generation Z. That the Generation Z, more liable to use the internet, attending to online survey more than other age groups is an indication of their being more liable to Internet-based transactions can be thought. It is normal that a generation, raised as acquainted with using the internet and social media, perceive online and offline as a perfect mixture (Chayko, 2018: 71). People being 37 years old and over with 27 %, people between 31 and 36 with 16 %, people between 19 and

Tab. 2: Internet Usage Info of Participants

Use of Internet		
Yes	379	99
No	3	1
Internet Use (Hour)		
Between 0–1 Hour	21	3
Between 2–4 Hours	196	51
Between 5–7 Hours	112	30
Between 8–10 Hours	37	10
12 Hours and Over	16	6

24 with 12 %, and finally people between 25 and 30 with 8 % have attended to the survey with a decreasing rate after the Generation Z. People born between years 1965 and 1980 are accepted as the Generation X. The Generation X both meet with the new inventions and innovation in their later lives and involved in the internet afterwards. Yet, the Generation X is the most attended group among people attending the online survey after the Generation Z. This shows that the internet is a technology used by all generations.

When the education levels of attendants are scrutinized, that 40 % are high school graduates is seen, and they are members of the Generation Z. That 38 % have bachelor's degrees is understood. People being high school graduates, having bachelor's degrees and continuing their education are the majority of attendants with 78 %.

Also, internet usage information is asked to the users. 99 % of 382 attendants state that they use the internet. That result shows that the internet is an inevitable part of our lives.

51 % of attendants express that they spend 2 or 4 hours on the internet daily. 30 % express that they spend between 5 and 7 hours on the internet daily. 10 % express that they spend 8 and 10 hours on the internet daily. When the internet use time is analyzed, connecting to the internet for between 2 and 4 hours daily is seen as quite ordinary. More than half of people attending the survey connect to the internet for at least 2 hours daily for whether work or just spending their free time. 6 % state that they use the internet for at least 12 hours daily. Also, 82 % of attendants state that they prefer to use their mobile phones to connect to the internet. From this point of view, mobile phones, including so many features such as communication, taking photos, video recording, music player, etc. are devices mostly preferred to connect to the internet. 9 % of attendants state that

Tab. 3: Ego-Surfing Information of Participants

Searching for their names		
Less than once in a month	341	89
Once in a month or three times	25	6
Once in a week	9	2
Two times or five times in a week	5	2
Once a day	2	1
Seeing my name makes me happy		
Absolutely agree	39	10
Agree	114	30
Undecided	104	28
Disagree	87	23
Absolutely not agree	38	9
Ego-surfing rate		
Yes	34	10
No	348	90

they prefer to use their portable computers to connect to the internet. As stated by Chayko, portability is the main feature of digital environment (2018: 43). In both cases, it is understood that connecting to the internet on the move is important for the users.

87 % of attendants choose the answer "no" among the choices given under the heading that I search for my name periodically on the internet, and they state that they do not exhibit this behavior. The rate of attendants, who exhibit the behavior of searching for their names periodically on the internet, showing the indications of online narcissism is 13 %. Although almost all the attendants express that they use the internet, 13 % exhibiting the behavior, called as ego-surfing, and them being connected to the internet do not mean that they absolutely have the behavior called as digital disorder.

Whereas 63 % of attendants express that they like their names, 89 % of people searching for their names on the internet express that they do that less than once in a month. This rate is another indication that most of the attendants do not ego-surf. The rate of people searching for their names once or three times in a month is 6 %, and the rate of people searching for their names once daily is 1 %, the lowest rate.

The definition of narcissism is explained to the attendants on the survey, and people are requested to describe themselves. That 24.5 % accept they see themselves as the narcissist and 75.5 % do not see themselves as narcissist is understood. However, 40 % of attendants express that they feel happy if they would see their names on the internet, and 33 % express that positive sharing about their names affect themselves. These data demonstrate that attendants are liable to ego-surf. The hormone of happiness called the serotonin is also effective on becoming addicted. People might be liable to perform the behaviors making themselves happy. In this context, if people search for their names on the internet and start to feel happy, they could start to ego-surf. 33 % of attendants express that they feel anxious if they do not look at the sharing and comments about themselves. Furthermore, 53 % of attendants express that negative comments about their names would affect themselves. Like happiness, anxiety is a factor causing people to have behaviors and it might create an effect which would lead to addictions.

The attendants are informed that ego-surfing is a digital disorder causing people to search for their names on the internet and follow the news about themselves periodically. Then the question of whether they think that they have this disorder or not is asked to the attendants. 90 % of attendants do not accept that they have it. However, 10 % express that they ego-surf and they feel happy when they do it. The rate of attendants, expressing that they search for their names on the internet, with 13 % is decreased after they are informed that this behavior is a digital disorder. Furthermore, 62 % of attendants express that they accept ego-surfing is an indication of narcissism. In this context, that the digital identities are also important for people, ego-surfing, might be asserted. As the statements, made about themselves in the virtual environment, being positive or negative affect their attitudes and behaviors in the real world.

Conclusion

Digital disorders, one of the digital disorders, ego-surfing, and its main reason, narcissism, are analyzed under the headings in this chapter. The deductions about how much the users are addicted and how often they search for their names on the internet are made in the chapter through the survey consisting of twenty questions. The internet has become an inevitable part of daily lives in the world. However, the overuse of internet, besides its positive sides such as searching for information, sharing information making trading easier, and being in contact with others, cause people to be addicted. According to the result of this research, of which sample consists of a group of 382 people randomly being reached to, almost all of attendants use the internet technologies routinely. That half of the attendants spare between 2 and 4 hours daily for internet use is understood. These data demonstrate that people spare at least two hours daily for internet use. When the time spent to connect to the internet is increased, that the possibility to become addicted might be increased is estimated. That people, called the Generation Z, are more apt to the digital world is acknowledged. This thought is approved after the attendants attending to the research are analyzed (37 % of attendants consist of people between 13 and 18 years old). And these are the members of the Generation Z. However, a remarkable result is that the group of attendants, being 37 years old and over with 27.4 %, are the most attended group after people of Generation Z. Although these people, called the Generation X, meet with the internet in their later life, they adapt themselves to the new technological channels and they use these actively.

That 13.6 % of attendants, to whom questions about their thoughts on online narcissism are asked, have this behavior is deduced from their expressions. However, this rate decreases to 9.3 % after the attendants are informed that searching for their own names on the internet periodically is an indication of disorder. This data demonstrate that the thoughts change when a behavior is considered as a disorder. The users searching for their names on the internet periodically and the ones who do this very frequently have almost the same information about this behavioral disorder, ego-surfing. Yet people do not have enough information about these disorders, showing up with technology addiction.

Online narcissism is one of the consequences of people becoming addicted to the internet. Ego-surfing is a digital behavioral disorder which people overusing the internet and social media might have. The users might search for their names frequently or periodically on the internet, and they might be happy when doing that. The reason behind of this is online narcissism. In online narcissism, the users like themselves, names and they become happy with positive post about themselves, and they become unhappy and uneasy because of the negative posts.

The deductions about how much the users are addicted and how often they search for their names are made in this chapter. Also, the demographic information, internet addiction, how much they see themselves as narcissistic, and how often people having online narcissism search for their names are tried to be determined by asking questions.

Furthermore, being active on social media, liking themselves too much, always looking at sharing about themselves, being happy by doing these, and being appreciated cause some satisfaction. This is a situation making people feel happy and most of them are unaware of the fact that this is a disorder.

Bibliography

Andreassen, C. S., Torsheim, T., Brunborg, G. S. & Pallesen, S. (2012). Development of a Facebook Addiction Scale, Psychological Reports, 110(2), 501–517. DOI: 10.2466/02.09.18.PR0.110.2.501-517.

Atkinson, R. L., Atkinson, R. C. & Hilgard, E. R. (1995). Psikolojiye Giriş (K. Atakay, M. Atakay & A. Yavuz, Trans.). İstanbul: Sosyal Yayınları.

Aziz, A. (2015). Araştırmanın Yazılması ve Sunulması, İstanbul: Hiperlink Yayınları.

Balcı, G. & Gülnar, B. (2009). Üniversite Öğrencileri Arasında İnternet Bağımlılığı ve İnternet Bağımlılarının Profili, Selçuk İletişim, 6(1), 5–22.

Başkurt, İ. (2003). Gençlik, Madde Bağımlılığı ve Korunma Yolları (Psiko-Sosyal Bir Yaklaşım), İstanbul Üniversitesi İlahiyat Fakültesi Dergisi, 8(2003), 73–114.

Bozkurt, H., Şahin, S. & Zoroğlu, S. (2016). İnternet Bağımlılığı: Güncel Bir Gözden Geçirme, Journal of Contemporary Medicine, 6(3), 235–247.

Buffardi, E. L. & Campbell, W. K. (2008). Narcissism and Social Networking Web sites. Personality and Social Psychology Bulletin, 34, 1303–1314. DOI:10.1177/0146167208320061.

Campbell, W. K., Rudich, E. A., & Sedikides, C. (2002). Narcissism, Self-Esteem, and the Positivity of Self-Views: Two Portraits of Self-Love. Personality and Social Psychology Bulletin, 28(3), 358–368.

Chayko, M. (2018). Süperbağlantılı-İnternet, Dijital Medya ve Tekno-Sosyal Hayat (B. Bayındır, D. Yengin & T. Bayrak, Trans.). İstanbul: Der Yayınları.

Coştu, Y. (2009). Toplumsallaşma Kavramı Üzerine Sosyolojik Bir Değerlendirme, Dinbilimleri Akademik Araştırma Dergisi, 9(3), 117–140.

Çam, E. & İşbulan, O. (2012). A New Addiction for Teacher Candidates: Social Networks, Turkish Online Journal of Educational Technology (TOJET), 11(3), 14–19.

Dinç, M. (2010). İnternet Bağımlılığı. İstanbul: Ferfir Yayınları.

Duygulu, S. (2017, August, 15). Teknoloji Bağımlılığı Hayatımıza E-Hastalıklar Olarak Girdi. Hürriyet Aile. Retrieved from http://www.hurriyetaile.com/yazarlar/serap-duygulu/internet-ve-sosyal-medya-hastaliklari-e-hastaliklar_6481.html on October 2017.

Düvenci, A. (2012). Ağ Neslinin Internet Kullanımı Üzerindeki Sosyal Medya Etkisinin Sosyal Sapma Yaklaşımı ile İncelenmesi (Doctoral dissertation). Marmara Üniversitesi, İstanbul, Türkiye.

Feldman, T. (1997). Introduction to Digital Media. London: Routledge.

Geray, H. (2003). İletişim ve Teknolojilerin Uluslararası Birikim Düzeninde Yeni Medya Politikaları. Ankara: Ütopya Yayınları.

Griffiths, M. D. (1998). Internet Addiction: Does it really exist? In J. Gackenbach (Ed.), Psychology and the Internet: Intrapersonal, Interpersonal and Transpersonal Applications (pp. 61–75). New York: Academic Press.

Gündüz, S. (2007). Health Problems with the Use of Information Technologies. Online Submission, Paper presented at the International Educational Technology (IETC) Conference (7th, Nicosia, Turkish Republic of Northern Cyprus)

Güngör, N. (2011). İletişim: Kuramlar ve Yaklaşımlar. Ankara: Siyasal Yayınları.

Hooper, V. & Zhou, M. (2007). Addictive, Dependent, Compulsive A Study of Mobile Phone Usage. 20th Bled eConference eMergence: Merging and Emerging Technologies, Processes, and Institutions (272–285). Bled, Slovenia.

Kandell, J. J. (1998). Internet Addiction on Campus: The Vulnerability of College Students, CyberPsychology & Behavior, 1(1), 11–17.

Kelleci, M. (2008). Internet, Cep Telefonu, Bilgisayar Oyunlarının Çocuk ve Gençlerin Ruh Sağlığına Etkileri. TAF Preventive Medicine Bulletin, 7(3), 253–256.

Kim, E. J., Namkoong, K., Ku, T., & Kim, S. J. (2008). The Relationship between Online Game Addiction and Aggression, Self-control and Narcissistic Personality Traits. European Psychiatry, 23(3), 212–218.

Köroğlu, E. & Bayraktar, S. (2007). Kişilik Bozuklukları. Ankara: HYB Yayınları.

Kurtaran, G.M. (2008). İnternet Bağımlılığını Yordayan Değişkenlerin İncelenmesi (Master's Thesis, Mersin Üniversitesi, Mersin, Turkey). Retrieved from https://tez.yok.gov.tr/UlusalTezMerkezi/tezSorguSonucYeni.jsp on 2 July 2018.

Kurtkan, A. (1979). Genel Sosyoloji. İstanbul: İstanbul Üniversitesi İktisat Fakültesi Yayıları.

Nalçaoğlu, H. (2003). Medya ve Toplum İlişkisini Anlamak Üzere Bir Çerçeve. In H. Nalçaoğlu & S. Alankuş (Eds.), Medya ve Toplum (pp. 43–57). İstanbul: IPS İletişim Vakfı Yayınları.

Ong, E. Y., Ang, R. P., Ho, J. C., Lim, J. C., Goh, D. H., Lee, C. S., & Chua, A. Y. (2011). Narcissism, Extraversion and Adolescents' Self-presentation on Facebook. Personality and Individual Differences, 50(2), 180–185.

Özsoy, T. (2009). Fastfood'dan Facebook'a: İnternet Bağımlılığı, Declaration of XI. Akademik Bilişim Conference 11–13 February 2009 Harran University, Şanlıurfa.

Öztürk, Ö., Odabaşıoğlu, G., Eraslan, D., Genç, Y. & Kalyoncu, Ö. A. (2007). İnternet Bağımlılığı: Kliniği ve Tedavisi. Bağımlılık Dergisi, 8(1), 36–41.

Polat, R. (2017). Dijital Hastalık Olarak Nomofobi. e-Journal of New Media, 1(2), 164–172.

Schumann, K. & Topçu, H. (2013, May 25). Dijital detoks. Deutsche Welle Türkçe. Retrieved from https://www.dw.com/tr/dijital-detoks/a-16836439 on 21 July 2015.

Suler, J. (1996). The Psychology of Cyberspace. Retrieved from http://www-usr.rider.edu/~suler/psycyber/supportgp.html on 24 January 2019.

Tarhan (2017, April 27). Kişi internetsiz ortamda krize giriyorsa bağımlılık başlamış demektir [Blogpost] Retrieved from https://www.nevzattarhan.com/prof-dr-nevzat-tarhan-kisi-internetsiz-ortamda-krize-giriyorsa-bagimlilik-baslamis-demektir.html.

Tarhan, N. & Nurmedov, S. (2013). Sanal veya Gerçek Bağımlılık. İstanbul: Timaş Yayınları.

T.C. Üsküdar Üniversitesi (2017). Prof. Dr. Nevzat Tarhan; "Gençler internette ego sörfü yapıyor". Retrieved from https://uskudar.edu.tr/tr/icerik/2053/prof-dr-nevzat-tarhan-gencler-internette-ego-sorfu-yapiyor on 26 Januar 2015.

Teknoloji 'e-hastalıkları' doğurdu (2017, March 2). Facebook depresyonu, ego sörfü, siberhondrik! T24.com.tr. Retrieved from http://t24.com.tr/haber/teknoloji-e-hastaliklari-dogurdu-facebook-depresyonu-ego-sorfu-siberhondrik,391625 on 5 December 2018.

Thurlow, C., Lengel, L. & Tomic, A. (2004). Computer Mediated Communication: Social Interaction and the Internet. London: Sage Publications.

Ulukol, B. (2013). Bilgi teknolojileri ve internetin bilinçli ve güvenli kullanımının sağlık boyutu. Retrieved from https://www.guvenliweb.org.tr/dosya/k1ve9.pdf on 10 December 2018.

Yengin, D. (2017). İletişim Çalışmalarında Araştırma Yöntemleri ve Uygulamaları. İstanbul: Der Yayınları.

Yurdagül, Ş. (1987). Bazı Sosyoekonomik Değişkenlerin Lise Öğrencilerinin Benlik Tasarımına Etkisi (Doctoral Dissertation). Turkey: Hacettepe Üniversitesi.

Hakan Tan

Digital Cynicism

Abstract: This chapter questions whether cynicism is also observed in digital space or not, based on behaviors and discourses of the individuals (actors) on some social media platforms they deal with. Does digital cynicism exist? Is digital cynicism a disorder that needs to be treated? What is normal, and what is abnormal? Is cynicism a dangerous philosophy for the society, or is it possible for it to have a positive function of stimulus for the society? The study, embracing these critical questions with nuances, discusses whether cynically fundamental behaviors and discourses are observed on some social media samples or not. The author questions whether cynicism, a highly special term in terms of its philosophical history, is experienced as digital cynicism today. In the study, some samples that display cynical behaviors without possibly not acting with the awareness of cynicism, i.e., unconsciously display them are interpreted.

Keywords: cynicism, digital cynicism, social influence, conformity, social media, self, compliance

Introduction

In the historical context, every society has a system of ideas and behaviors that are provided by a certain norm, morality, value and social consensus. The person adapts the behavior of the family, work, group, community and society in which he/she lives, communicates and cooperates in the environment and the scene he/she lives (e.g., in social media). The definition of conformity by people is explained by social psychology with the following concepts: compliance, identification and internalization. However, social sciences examine the processes of interaction; the participation of individuals within the communities and societies; and the effects of processes on individuals, communities and societies. The leading concepts in the development of the social sciences are as follows: positivism for Comte; organism for Spener; anomie, division of labor, transition between lower and upper structures and structures of society for Durkheim (2012, 2014a, 2014b); economy, society, religion and capitalism for Weber (2012a, 2012b, 2013); for Parsons, adopting Weberian ideas and combining with Durkheimian view, according to many thinkers, adapting the information, knowledge and cybernetic societies to the society (1968) "adaptation", "goal", "attainment", "integration" and "latency". These concepts are abbreviated as "A.G.I.L." by Parsons (Mattelart, 2004; Güngör, 2013; Vanderstraeten, 2012).

Talcott Parsons considers the individual as an actor and the actor pursues the goals. The actor is active, has roles and status. Actors are active in the social system. Parsons classifies the systems as cultural, personal and organic, and the relationship between systems is provided in a hierarchical context of information and cybernetic control. Habermas (1996), an influencer of the critical approach argues that the concepts of agreement, conflict, dialogue, and reconciliation, by benefiting from the A.G.I.L asserted by Talcott Parsons, can take place in the rational public environment (Yavaşgel, 2014). According to the intellectuals, who examine society as a system of behaviors and thoughts, individuals are actors that play their roles on a stage within a certain classification and division of labor. The actor has the norm, law, morality and values to comply with. While Durkheim defines the actors that do not play their roles as anomie (normlessness, derangement), Goffman, who carries out the studies within the framework of Mead's ideas, considers the individuals as actors, similarly to Parsons, and explains the performance of the person and the fact that the person is convinced of the reality of his/her act by the concept of "sincerity". According to Goffman, a cynical performer is one who "may be moved to guide the conviction of this audience only as a means to other ends, having no ultimate concern about the values and beliefs of the audience". According to Goffman, a cynical individual *"may experience an unprofessional pleasure from his/her own deception by acting professionally distanced; or experience spiritual aggression as the cynical individual is glad to be able to play as s/he wishes with something that the audience takes seriously"* (Goffman, 2014).

The first person to outline the cynicism is Antisthenes, first a pupil of sophist Gorgias and then of Socrates. The cynicism is both influenced by the "return to nature" idea of Hippias and Euripides and the Socrates' philosophy on life (interrogation, to become self-sufficient, the significance of the moral knowledge, virtue, integrity, etc.) Although the classic cynics, who are the representatives of the Cynic school of thought, are interested in daily life communication (environment/scene), interaction and cooperation with other people, they did not conform with the group, community and the society. Diogenes Laertios, who lived 600 years after Antisthenes said, *"In life, you were a dog Antisthenes (...) As to bite the heart with words, not with the mouth!"* about him. (Laertios, 2017: 259). The behavior of people, who behave abnormally in Ancient Greece is called cynic, which means dogs to them because the behaviors are compared to the dog. Cynics do not take offense when people call them "dogs"; however, they exalt the concept of cynicism.

Michel Foucault draws attention to the importance of examining the subject, personality, power relations and the behavior of the person in his works

(1995, 2008, 2015a, 2015b, 2015c, 2015d, 2015e, 2016). Michel Foucault states that people in the Middle Ages have considered abnormal people as patients, but that this is only limited with *"a few people" and that particularly an industrial society has been formed and that these abnormal people are no longer allowed (Foucault, 2015a: 162–163; Foucault, 2015e; 79).* Furthermore, Foucault (2015e; 21) refers to the separation and rupture of the distance between the mind and the non-minded and emphasizes the importance of talking about the wholeness of the contemporary mind to be able to speak about the gap. Today's people, society and the structures created by the society (such as science, jurisdiction, executive, legislative bodies and economy) can explain the behavior of classical cynics as crime, disease and madness. According to Foucault, there are three reasons behind it: a) medical thought, b) social norms created by power relations and , c) people's willingness to conform to society. Because, according to Michel Foucault, "medical thought is about separating the normal from the abnormal" and, moreover, people adapting to society and living by the norms constitute "one of the greatest power devices of the contemporary society" (Foucault, 2015a: 156–157).

Foucault's research is based on power techniques and power technology. The principal part of his research is about how power lead people to obey by applying domination with the techniques and technologies that the power possesses (Foucault, 2015a: 246). Foucault connects the conformity of social psychology that is represented by the obedience, to the techniques and technology of the power (Foucault, 1995, 2015a, 2015b, 2015c, 2015d, 2015e, 2016). On the other hand, Foucault *says "there is no society without rules, there is no society without a restrictive system; there is no natural society as it is widely known"* (Foucault, 2015a: 216). Therefore, in the historical context, there is a system of behavior in every society that renders a certain norm and social compromise. According to Foucault, individuals in contemporary societies conform to society and social structures from the framework of norms, criteria and constraints created by power relations, society, social structures and capitalism. Therefore, those who do not conform to the norms, moral values and constraints created by the power relations, society, social structures and capitalism can be defined as criminals, patients and insane. According to Foucault, the person who is excluded for power relations and capitalism "is *the person who needs to be improved to be included in the system*" (Foucault, 2015a: 233). This study aims to answer the following questions, " Can we consider the cynicism as a disease?" or "Can we consider a cynic as a person that needs to be improved so that the person can be included in the society and social structures?". When examining the Turkish literature, there is no article found that describes the relationship between digital and social media and cynicism. The actors are defined as "cynic" if they do not accept the social role in a media, in a scene or in an environment; do not conform to the social influence; do not conform to the norms and do not accept the social role; express his/her thoughts freely; strive to explain the truth, honesty and reality; do not take into consideration the social values, thoughts and behaviors; and show a cynical or aggressive attitude to the rules of social norm, morality, value, manners and discipline. The concepts of stage, role and actor are frequently used by ego-theorists.

In the studies of William James, G. Herbert Mead (2017) and Erving Goffman in terms of ego-theory (1978) emphasize the concepts of the stage, actor, role and theater. According to Mead, the mind is shaped by symbols, which are elements of the science of communication and the ego is formed by the process of communication and interaction with others and objects in the life of the person. *"According to Mead, ego is an actor"* (Wallace & Wolf, 2015: 276). *"For Mead, the ego constitutes a social structure in essence and it is formed within the social structure"* (Habermas, 1996: 466). The person's ego is formed during a process of communication, interaction and cooperation with others and objects that exist in the life of the person. Goffman also concentrates on the notion of the actor as Mead does. In the study called "The Presentation of Self in Everyday Life", Goffman (1978) stated people act in daily life when expressing themselves, sometimes strive to deceive other people, and they benefit from a set, stage and scene for displaying their performance. *"As Goffman indicates, social interactions often involve "a staging of the ego", in which everyone seeks to adopt and maintain a respectable image of himself/herself, considered as the social identity"* (Bourse and Yücel, 2012: 269). According to Goffman, the self is a dramatic result that is presented on the stage. On the other hand, social media is a scene as well.

The desire of the people to socialize and the opportunity provided by the technology created the social media channels and verified the concept of "Global Village", used by McLuhan and Powers (1992). In traditional media, people that are readers, listeners and viewers can participate in social media; in other words, they can take a part on stage through the characteristics of interaction, participation and sharing. In social media, the sender and the receiver perform a shared and interactive communication via the same channel (media/environment). Hence, the sender and the receiver can be both active and passive in this communication environment (Tan, 2017a; Tan, 2017b). Mediated communication (media) is transformed into an unmediated communication, thanks to the technological possibilities. The mimics, gestures, body language, images and the meanings of them that are emphasized by Mead and Goffman are also very prominent in social media. Kaplan and Haenlein (2010) highlight that social media creates a visual social world, which increases the possibilities for the presentation of the self. People can present their selves on social media by technological possibilities; in other words, they are actors who play their roles on a stage. It is possible that the actors that are related to social media in terms of cynicism can act in the following ways: a) they do not participate in social media, b) do not share anything although they are subscribed, or ending their subscription in the social media after a while so that they do not conform to the social influence, c) share something without taking into consideration the social values, morality and social ideas although they are subscribed to the social media and d) they participate in social media but as Diogenes Laertius emphasizes, "I tell the ugliest truth to the bad, liar people and reveal the truth about them (...) *Other dogs bite their enemies, I bite my friends to save them*". As they are opposed to some data, findings and information, they focus on how to achieve the knowledge and virtue. They can present their selves, their roles, their behaviors and thoughts through sharing, participation and interactions and telling the truth.

Cynicism-Cynic Concepts and Cynic School

Cynicism (Fr. Cynisme; Gr. Zynismus) is expressed as "Sinisizm", "Sinizm" and "Sinik" in Turkish. In the dictionary of Turkish Language Association (TDK) the term "Sinik" is explained as intimidated, frustrated and frightened. The term "Sinik" does not provide the meaning of ideas, daily behaviors and the expressions of the thought, which are touched upon in cynicism philosophy and by the supporters of this philosophy; thus the terms "kinizm" and "kinik" are used in this study.

"*Cynicism is at first a school of thought of sophist Gorgias then a school of thought of Antisthenes, who is a pupil of Socrates. It is also influenced by both "return to nature" idea of Hippias and Euripides and the Socrates' philosophy on life (interrogation, to become self-sufficient, the significance of the moral knowledge, virtue, integrity, etc.) The essence of the philosophy of cynicism is that person can reach himself/herself by virtue and happiness, independent from all necessities, regardless of value*" (Cevizci, 2017: 1138). Diogenes Laertius, in his work called "Lives and Opinions of Eminent Philosophers" (3rd century AC), mentions his efforts to become a student of Socrates and Antisthenes and to listen to the lectures of Socrates. It is explained by the philosophers that Socrates praises Antisthenes at the end of various events. In his work "A Dog's Luck", Georg Luck (2011) describes the philosophy of cynicism in Antiquity, the foundation of the Cynic School and the persons, who expanded the Cynic discipline. According to Luck, the most immediate influence for the Cynic school was Socrates (Luck,

2011: 16). Antisthenes, a pupil of Socrates, is the founder of the Cynic School with his lifestyle and discipline (Arslan, 2017: 157; Timuçin, 2004: 323; Luck, 2011: 47; Diogenes, 2017: 252). Laertius Diogenes describes the essence of Antisthenes' doctrine as follows: *"Only virtuous people are noble; the virtue is necessary to attain happiness and virtue does not need anything other than the power of Socrates"* (Laertios, 2017: 255). Antisthenes based his doctrine on virtue and being virtuous like Socrates. On the other hand, Antisthenes states, *"The wise man would regulate his conduct, not according to the established law of the state, but according to the law of virtue".* According to Socrates, the virtuous person is wise, and knowledge also determines the behavior of the person. Hence, Socrates has spent the rest of his life searching for information at all costs and questioned unceasingly the correctness and source of knowledge. According to Socrates, *"'knowing thyself' (gnothi seauton) is related to knowing the person, taking care of thyself and the care of self (epimelia heautou)". In other words, it is the ability of the person to dominate thyself.* (Foucault, 2015c: 5).

On the other hand, Plato (2014), in his book called *The Defence of Socrates*, explains that Socrates draws attention to the significance of living in a society by obeying the rules of ethics, norms, morals and laws throughout his life. In addition, Plato explains that Socrates emphasizes the necessity and importance of individuals, particularly administrators, to conform to ethics, norms, morality and laws under every circumstance. Although Socrates told the truth, he was sentenced to death by the Athenian Council. Many prominent figures of Athens encouraged Socrates to flee. However, he refused to flout the law and escape his legal responsibility and Socrates executed his death sentence. According to Kalayci (2015), although Socrates told the truth, he was sentenced to death by the Athenian Council. That is why Antisthenes and his followers (cynics) do not conform to the social contract, social manners, social laws and social moral values that are highly emphasized by Socrates and for which, Socrates risked his life. *The death sentence of Socrates was legal, but not fair.* (Kalayci, 2015: 81). Kalaycı, therefore, emphasizes that cynics consider laws (nomos) and political civilization (bios and police) as a problem. Kalaycı states that cynics exhibit their roles, their selves, their thoughts and behaviors in an environment and on the stage within the framework of the following approach, *"They do not follow social rules, they exceed the limits of manners, they do not obey the law, they reject the comfort and finally, they adopt a natural way of life".* On the other hand, Arslan reveals that the Cynic School is separated from Socrates' doctrine at this point and according to the cynics, the virtue signifies a practical application, rather than the knowledge (Arslan, 2017: 163). Although cynics engage in communication, interaction and cooperation with other people in everyday life (environment/

scene), they do not tend to conform to the rules of the groups, community and society. Therefore, Diogenes Laertius quotes a reference to Antisthenes: *"In life, you were a dog, Antisthenes (…) As to bite the heart with words, not with the mouth!"* (Laertius, 2017: 259). People thought Antisthenes, the founder of the Cynic school of thought, lived like a dog in Ancient Greece because he did not conform to the social behavior and social systems of thought, such as the dominant social norms, moral values and forms of politeness in Ancient Greece. Since the way Antisthenes expresses his life and thoughts is defined as a dog by other people, the followers of cynicism philosophy, discipline and school are called the "cynic".

The name "Cynic" derives from Ancient Greek word of "Kyon" (dog). People who support cynicism are called cynics (Eng. Cynics; French Cyniques; German Kyniker/Zyniker). People who exhibit their thoughts and behaviors in the cynicism discipline are called the "kyon" in Greek because their lifestyles are similar to the lives of dogs. One of the leading figures of cynicism is Diogenes (412–323 BC), who is born in Sinop. *"Diogenes is the person who approached the most to the words 'cynic' or 'dog' with his lifestyle"* (Timuçin, 2014: 323). Cynics do not take offense when people call them "dogs"; however, they exalt the concept of cynicism. For example, Diogenes explained to the people who asked why he is called a dog as following, *"Because I tell the truth to the liar and bad people and I tell the truth about themselves. I flick my tail to the good people, but I growl at bad people". In another case, Diogenes said, "Other dogs bite their enemies, I bite my friends to save them"*. The most important thing for cynics is the *"freedom and independence"* (Arslan, 2017: 164). It is told that "*Plato describes Diogenes as a Socrates gone mad*" (Luck, 2011: 16). According to Diogenes, the most beautiful thing in the world is the *"freedom of speech"* (Laertius, 2017: 279; Luck, 2011: 131). According to the Internet Encyclopedia of Philosophy, the most important thing for cynics is freedom and they advocate the freedom in three forms: eleutheria (liberty), autarkeia, (self-sufficiency) and parrhēsia, (freedom of speech). Cynics question the lives and thoughts of others in the society, in which they live freely, according to a Socratic approach; they believed that in order to attain virtue and being virtuous, they should express their opinions freely, at any cost. In addition, cynics expressed their thoughts in everyday life (temples, baths, shops and street corners), not in a school, as other schools did, so that the school becomes popular. They also demonstrated their thoughts with their behavior; in other words, cynics expressed their teachings in their daily life practices.

The cynics literally lived like dogs. "*Diogenes ate raw meat and didn't use the fire. Cynics could fulfil their physical needs (lovemaking, pee, etc.) where they eat*" (Kalaycı, 2015: 83). For example, Crates and his wife Hipparchia, who adopted the Cynic philosophy, abandoned all their wealth and social status, lived like a dog and also had sex in public (Luck, 2011: 231). Ethical laws of society, social conventions, social behavior patterns and the obedience of the other persons in society in these rules can prevent the virtuous life for Cynics. Therefore, these values are considered *"absurd and ridiculous"* by Cynics (Cynics, n.d.). Cynics rejected fame, nobility, pleasure, social discipline, manners, rules and laws. They opposed social behavior and did not conform to or adopt social rules. This situation is not found acceptable in Antiquity as the philosophers also stated. It is obvious that some people today will not be welcomed by the social, juridical and cultural traditions, rules, rules of manners and laws if they would live as the classical cynics lived in Antiquity. In fact, this situation can be defined as madness, crime and disease. On the other hand, cynicism is a choice and act. The act is explained as a decision in thought while it is behavior in action.

Discussion: On the Concept of Cynicism

As Foucault emphasizes, today's world may explain the behaviors of cynics as a crime, disease and madness. For example, according to the study by Şimşek (2015), *"cynicism (...) is an organizational chronic disease, of which the treatment isn't found yet"* (Şimşek, 2015: 254). Cynicism has been examined in the Turkish literature so far as to be more organizational and consumeristic. (Yalçınkaya, 2014; Candan, 2013; Argon and Ekinci, 2016; Karacaoğlu and İnce, 2012; Üçok and Torun, 2014; Kart, 2015, Odou and Pechpeyrou, 2011; Güven, 2016; Boush et al., 1993). In organizational studies, the actor's performance is measured by the *"efficiency"*. The reason of the organizational cynicism is explained by the fact that the actor does not believe in and trust the words or the managers, the justice in the work environment, the principles of equality or if the employment brings any benefit or if they would be included in decision-making processes and organizational policies. The actor's performance in consumeristic studies is measured by *"consuming"*. In consumption cynicism, for example, according to Odou and Pechpeyrou, *four types of cynicism are described: a) defensive, b) offensive, c) subversive and d) ethical (Odou ve Pechpeyrou, 2011: 1801).* According to Odou and Pechpeyrou, the "defensive cynic" avoids being deceived by the image and persuasion activities for the proper interests of the brands; while the "offensive cynic" strives to look out for own interests. The "subversive cynic" supports the deciphering of the consumption code that provides the consumer ideology and strongly condemns this hegemony while the "ethical cynic" master's one's own life by casting off the artificial and natural chains. According to Güven (2016), the reasons for the consumeristic cynicism are, *"perception of being used by a company; unmet expectations; deceptiveness of advertising messages; need to develop defensive mechanisms; the need for persons to be able to control their own lives"* (Güven, 2016: 163). Therefore, if the actors work efficiently on the stage (the business environment) and adopt the norm, rule, working conditions of the organization, play the internalized roles and consume high rates and accept advertising messages; they become part of the production and consumption society, they behave normally. In addition, according to studies on cynicism, there is a consensus that cynicism represents a cognitive, emotional and behavioral negative attitude (Güven, 2016: 152; Üçok and Torun, 2014: 231; Karacaoğlu and İnce, 2012: 78). Therefore, in order to prevent the negative situations that cynic people would cause on other people, to improve and persuade the cynics, the brand and business management should make activities. As social scientists emphasize, today's people act as actors within the social system. In order to accept the actors as normal, it is expected that they will adopt the norms and laws created by the thought and behavior systems within the social system, obey them and even act like actors in a scene after being identified within the system.

On the other hand, in order for people to feel insecure in social (family, friends, etc.), business, economy and political environments; to think, to behave and to question the system of social, global thoughts and behaviors; the information must be emerged at first. If we refer to Diogenes, it is necessary to be cynical for saying the truth, for protecting his friends and biting his enemies. For example, Julian Bagnini's news in "The Guardian" about the former American intelligence employee, Edward Snowden, can be cited as an example (Baggini, 2013). In the case, later filmed, Snowden revealed that the National Security Agency (NSA) of, the US cyber intelligence agency surveilled the whole world, (particularly USA), via the Internet, mobile phones and social media (Aytekin, 2018). In the article in "The Guardian", Baggini said, *"it is time to reclaim cynicism for the forces of light and truth"* (Baggini, 2013). On the other hand, as it is widely known, the US declared Snowden a traitor and Snowden had to seek asylum in Russia. With an analogy to Socrates, the trial and conviction of Snowden are in accordance with American law, but this is unfair. Snowden can be declared as guilty of explaining truth and reality in honesty.

After Cambridge Analytica, the business partner of Facebook revealed that data from millions of Facebook users were used, Edward Snowden declared Facebook as an "accomplice", not the "victim". Snowden recalled that in 2016, Cambridge Analytica, a company that collected data from 50 million Facebook users in 2014, collaborated with Facebook on the election campaign of US Presidential candidate Donald Trump (T24, 2018). On the other hand, according to the news of Digitalage, CIA can control the microphone and cameras of targeted computers and smartphones (Kutsal, 2017). Personal information, voices, pictures, shopping habits, visited locations of the *"normal"* individuals that conform to the social influence can be learned by hackers, intelligence organizations and brand management. Cynics expressing truth, reality and liberation warn the society about the stage, in which the persons demonstrate the behaviors that conform to the social influence. The concepts of cynicism and cynic philosophy, which is a concept of antiquity, are now being used on the Internet, new media and social media environments that work with the digital code.

Social Influence: Concepts of Compliance, Identification and Internalization

The person tends to conform to the family, business environment, group, community, society, stage (e.g., new and social media), in which he/she communicates, interacts, cooperates and shares. Arkonaç (2016) states that there are two concerns about conformity behavior: *"First of all, people want to make sure that what they think, their actions, their feelings and what they feel is right and appropriate; secondly, people avoid that other people have negative thoughts about them and want to create a good impression on other people"* (Arkonaç, 2016: 208–214). Social psychology also examines the behavior of family, group, community and society in a person's life, and analyses the factors that affect the conformity behavior in three categories: environmental, personal and cultural factors. Conformity behavior is explained with the concepts of "compliance", "identification" and "internalization" (Kağıtçıbaşı and Cemalcılar, 2015; İnceoğlu, 2011; Arkonaç, 2016). Factors affecting conformity behavior are presented in Tab. 1. According to Tab. 1, the factors that affect the conformity behavior of a person can be described as following: social media relations, the size of the group (the penetration into social media is rapidly increasing), being face to face (through new media and social media technology, that transforms into an intermediated communication), adherence to the group (the dependency on new and social media becomes the research subject of communication discipline), the formation, acquisition, development, presentation and loss of the ego. The size of the group and the importance of the group for the individual greatly affect the individual's compliance with the group. Since the group allows the individual's ego to develop, get nourished and to be presented (identification), s/he presents his/her ego (image management) and wants to direct others' behaviors by controlling them (image/communication management). The process of compliance and identification leads to the individual's adoption of the environment, space and scene in the framework of pragmatist thinking (utilitarianism).

Tab. 1: Factors Affecting Conformity Behavior. (Source: Kağıtçıbaşı and Cemalcılar, 2015: 78)

Environmental Factors	Personal Factors	Cultural Factors
1) Size of the Social Group	1) Effects of the Self	1) Individualistic and Collectivist Culture
2) Concurrence among Group Members	2) Need of Being an Individual	
3) Status and Prestige	3) Desire for Personal Control	
4) Face-to-face Communication	4) Effect of the Competence	
5) Loss of Self	5) Gender	
6) Commitment to the Group		
7) Commitment to the Interaction in the Future		
8) Effect of the Minority		

Compliance, identification and internalization concepts were first distinguished by Kelman (1961) (Kağıtçıbaşı and Cemalcılar, 2015: 95; İnceoğlu, 2011: 125). Therefore, the compliant person is passive and the person conforms to the social influence. Consequently, the compliance is *"the conformity behaviour without evaluating anything, just acting this way because other people ask the individual to or the other people act this way and that signifies changing the behaviour by complying to something"*(Ertürk, 2017: 53; Arkonaç, 2016: 26). In identification behavior, the person is active but not conscious. One feels like the others, mimicking the other person/persons by imitating, taking the model and acting. In addition, the behavior that the individual identifies should have a value for the individual. *"So identification is the adoption of the characteristics of the admired person"* (Ertürk, 2017: 54). On the other hand, if this admiration for the person is lost (the respect disappears), the person does not maintain the identification behavior. In the internalization behavior, the person is active and conscious. The person is aware of the benefits provided by the behavior he/she conforms to, and the person fits him/herself because he/she certainly believes that the behavior is appropriate and valuable (Güney, 2012; Ertürk, 2017; Kağıtçıbaşı and Cemalcılar, 2015). According to Kağıtçıbaşı and Cemalcılar, the first stage of conformity behavior against social influence consists of the compliance, the second stage is the identification and the last stage is internalization. According to Güney (2012), Ertürk (2017) and İnceoğlu (2011), the benefits of exhibiting "compliance", "identification" and "internalization" are as follows: being accepted, rewarded, not being punished, ensuring the self-development, being fulfilled emotionally, satisfying the needs of love, displaying creativity, being admired, being like someone, who is appreciated and the wish of the individual to do the right thing. People can participate in social media; share visual and auditory signs; and interact, collaborate and communicate with others in order to benefit from the advantages of compliance, identification and internalization.

Relationship between Social Media and the Self

Through the development of the Internet and technology, convergence and digitization have created new media by the means of communication. The desire of people to socialize and the opportunities of technology have created the social media channels by verifying McLuhan's concept of "global village". The individuals participate in social media by either complying or identifying themselves and conform to the social influence. According to the results of the survey conducted by "We Are Social" in 2018, 3.196 billion people, representing 42 % of the world's population, participate in social media channels. The participation rate in social media channels in Turkey is 63 % of the population. The number of Facebook users in Turkey is 51 million. When ranking the users in proportion to the population in the world, Turkey is the second country to penetrate Instagram (We Are Social, 2018). People with social influence participate in social media to show compliance within the group. The factors that affect people to conform, as emphasized in the section "social influence", are as follows: a) the idea of creating a good impression; and b) the need to make sure that his/her thoughts, actions, emotions and things that s/he feels are correct and appropriate.

According to Fuchs, *"social media and web 2.0 terms have been popular in recent years to explain the varieties of WWW applications such as microblogs such as blogs, Twitter, social networking sites, video/image/file sharing platforms, and wikis"* (Fuchs, 2016: 49). On the other hand, Tasner explains, *"the term of Web 2.0 as a collaboration, blogging, content sharing, online video sharing, social networking while Web 3.0 signifies mobile browsing, live video broadcasting, microblogging, personalization, and semantic terms"* (Tasner, 2011: 19). With the technologic possibilities expand, Fuchs and Tasner emphasize that people can produce and share content in social media, and they are in interaction, cooperation and communication. Through the social media, people can do the following: they are looking for a job, meeting other people, accessing information, setting up friendship groups, uploading the videos to social media so that the other people can watch, communicating news to thousands or even millions of people through microblogs. In addition, in social media networks, such as Facebook, Wikipedia,

Myspace, Twitter, YouTube, Instagram and Pinterest, people can share their thoughts, tastes, wishes, curiosities and perceptions voluntarily, and learn about the thoughts, wishes, desires, curiosities and perceptions of others. Thanks to the characteristics of Web 2.0 and 3.0, the individuals can send their liking and access them.

The concept of self is described as knowledge, beliefs, and thoughts about who, what and what characteristics and our efforts to create and present the self, also as strategies of impression management and self-presentation, and these efforts are characterized as "the war of being" (Kağıtçıbaşı and Cemalcılar, 2015: 248; Ertürk, 2011: 74; Ertürk, 2017: 122). One must be a member of a community for the formation, development and nourishment of the self, and needs to adopt the attitude of the "generalized other", as emphasized by Mead. Accordingly, the self is closely related to social structure, social behavior and social experience. In this way, the self is formed by the process of common attitudes and the person is gaining the self. The self consists of experiences, relationships, cooperation, participation, sharing and interaction with others – in other words, symbolic systems, behavioral systems and technology. It is the ability of the self to realize the self from the outside and to see the self as an object. In the development, nutrition and realization of the self; the symbol, the gesture, the experience, the subject, the body, our extensions, the other people, the objects, the memories, the people's desire to have awareness and superiority over others are very prominent. Consequently, there is a need for a scene, other people, social structure, nature and/or images produced by the human being for the formation, development and nutrition of the self.

According to Goffman, the self is a dramatic result that is presented on the stage. Social media also provides a scene (environment) for the formation, development and nurturing of the self, which enables individuals to express their selves and a group for the interaction of the self with others. Through social media, people are able to realize their selves, to reach out to others' comments about themselves, to adopt the attitudes of others, and to go through compliance, identification and internalization processes in order to communicate with the social structure and the generalized others.

Cynicism on Digital and Social Media

The article is written in Istanbul Aydın University within the context of the doctoral dissertation called "Transformation of Personal and Brand Image Management in Social Media". The article aims to examine the relationship between the concept of cynicism and the social media, which is a scene in which people can demonstrate their behavior, and how cynics, in other words, actors (examples of cynic behavior) present themselves in social media (they present their selves). This article provides the details about the historical origins of cynicism and current cynic approach, questions, whether cynicism is a disease, a negative thought and behavior, or it is a thought or behavior that needs to be improved. The answers to these questions are sought, benefiting from the works and researches of philosophers and the relationship between the cynicism and the concepts of social media and self, as emphasized by Goffman as well. In this article, the observation method is used by using the documents as Duverger (2014: 117–137) stated with descriptive research method among the communication research methods. The article is remarkable in terms of searching the answer to the question of whether the concept of cynicism is a disease and in terms of establishing the relationship between digital, new and social media and cynicism, and demonstrating that cynicism is exhibited in social media.

The performance of the actor in social media can be explained as *"producing, consuming and producing what you consume"*. In other words, the person becomes a member/participant, communicates with and interacts with the other people and brands, and displays the images (visual, auditory, conceptual) of his/her activity and the places he/she performs while consuming and living. Social media is a scene like the classic cynics expose their thoughts and behaviors in *daily life* (at the stage-temple, baths, shops and street corners). *It is a scene like the cynics present, express and exhibit their self, thoughts, and behaviors.* It is possible that the actors that are related to social media in terms of cynicism can act in the following ways: (a) they do not participate in social media, (b) do not share anything although they are subscribed, or ending their subscription in the social media after a while so that they do not conform to the social influence, (c) share something without taking into consideration the social values, morality and social ideas although they are subscribed to the social media, (d) they participate in social media but as Diogenes Laertius emphasizes, *"I tell the ugliest truth to the bad, liar people and reveal the truth about them (...) Other dogs bite their enemies, I bite my friends to save them"*. As they are opposed to some data, findings and information, they focus on how to achieve the knowledge and virtue. They can present their selves, their roles, their behaviors and thoughts through sharing, participation and interactions and telling the truth.

Jothimani et al. (2015) examine the students, who do not participate in social networking sites and discontinue the relationship with social media, with the interpretive structural modelling (ISM), although social networking sites allow people to share text, visual and video, and transform the social life. Researchers are investigating the reasons for the attitudes and behaviors of actors that act like mentioned in the headings a) and b) above in terms of the relationship between social media and the cynicism. In this study, they investigate the reasons why students do not participate in social media and the reasons why they discontinue the relationship with social media. In other words, the reasons of the students for not participating in social media even though they are subscribed to social media, even they end their subscriptions to social media after a while by not conforming to the social influence. According to the results of the research, it is determined that the students have a poor academic performance and the social media accounts are disabled by fear of losing opportunities during Placement. The lowest factors constitute the attack of multiple computers on an IP and cyberbullying. It is comprehended that the sample in the study has low economic income and comes from another country. On the other hand, students are aware of the dangers of cyberbullying and the IP that belongs to them. In addition, individuals have many tools and scenes for the formation and development of their selves except for social media.

Goffman uses the concept of "sincerity" for the individuals adopting their roles and performing while he explains the contrary situation by "cynicism". Goffman (1978, 2014) describes the characteristics of cynicism in five headings: a) A cynic actor does not care about the beliefs and values of the audience, b) A cynical performer can direct the beliefs of the audience only to achieve other purposes, c) A cynic performer can be emotionally aggressive by getting pleasure from something that the audience takes seriously, d) A cynic actor can take an unprofessional pleasure from his/her deceptive behaviors and from his/her own deception, e) A cynic actor does not believe in the role s/he plays and is not fascinated by the role s/he plays. In Tab. 2, the relationship between the characteristics of the cynicism indicated by Goffman and social media is examined through the content shared on social media, and the examples shared in traditional and digital media. On the other hand, it is not examined whether the people in the news examined in social media samples are a cynic. According to Tab. 2, the characteristics of the cynicism that Goffman mentions are realized on social media.

In Tab. 2, it is comprehended that the characteristics of the cynicism that Goffman stated were realized in the news reflected on digital, new and social media. The actors have a cynical approach to the behaviors mentioned by Goffman in the article a) and c) in terms of the characteristics of cynicism. In addition, the actors do not value the historical, cultural and political images, customs, norms, values, beliefs, and perceptions that are owned by the persons forming the society and social structures, and it is comprehended from social media that even these actors are happy to be able to treat these values like this. When the intellectual, historical and religious values, norms, ethics, signs, images

Tab. 2: Realization of Cynic Characteristics as Goffman Mentions in Social Media

Characteristics of Cynicism	Social Media Examples	Analysis
a) A cynic actor does not care about the beliefs and values of the audience.	(Blog sözlük, 2017) It is seen in the video that the person sits on the Atatürk's bust and has a cynical approach.	Although the person said that s/he knew that s/he was against the conformity, behavior, rules and norms that prevail in the society by sitting on the bust of Atatürk; s/he said that s/he was sitting on the bust of Atatürk because s/he likes Atatürk and s/he is talking to Atatürk. The person praises some actors in today's political life while criticizing some other actors and ends the video by saying some negative sentences that the society and norms will not approve about the actors s/he does not like.
	(Fama Haber, 2017) There is a video that a person shares on the social media channels during the New Year's Eve. There was a great reaction in the society after the video was viewed by people and this news was largely shown in the national news channels and it was widely discussed in the political environment.	While explaining some of his negative thoughts about the country he lives in at the New Year's Eve in 2017, he talks about the beliefs and values of some sections of the society in a cynical way. Some people in the community, who viewed the video, want to punish the person on his return to the country, considering that the content of the video was wrong according to their beliefs and values. The political authority on the events occurred emphasizes that the people in the society cannot punish the person concerned and that this should be done by law, rules and norms and the rights of the person should be defended.
	(Barlas, 2017) It is explained that the person shares a visual with the toy penis and gets the reactions via Instagram.	According to the report of Sözcü newspaper, the person (underaged singer) that has 1.3 million followers on Instagram shared a photo, and there is a toy penis on it. This was noticed by the parents of this singer's admirers, and this person gets highly negative reactions. According to the report, the person does not care about the beliefs and values of the society and the values of the parents. According to the news, this photo is not accepted by medical science either.

Tab. 2: (continued)

Characteristics of Cynicism	Social Media Examples	Analysis
b) A cynical player can direct the beliefs of the audience only to achieve other purposes,	(Ulus, 2017) There is a news about a mother blogger with 200,000 followers. The father files a lawsuit against his wife, claiming that the mother wants to gain a reputation by sharing images of the children on social media.	According to the news, the mother who has two children is filed to the court on the allegation that the children have been used in advertising on social media, and there was a child abuse and the court justifies the father. Experts also explain that this decision of the court may establish a precedent. According to the news, the person wants to make money by using the beliefs, values, habits and practices of the audience in social media to make the advertisements of the products. Therefore, according to the news, the mother may lose custody of her children by law.
	("Paylaşımlarıyla tepki çeken öğretmen", 2018) There is news of a person, who is fired because he had negative comments on social media about the girls, who participate in a physical education lesson.	According to the news the person says, "if the girls wear a tracksuit, they look naked" and shares this on social media according to his beliefs. As there are many negative reactions to this statement, the person is fired from the Ministry of Education. According to the news, it is comprehended that the person wants to direct, inform and convince social media viewers in accordance with his beliefs and values.
	("Sosyal medyanın en", 2017) A person can share naked images on social media and on the Internet.	According to the news, people who want to be famous and celebrity share their naked photos on social media channels, and they can receive positive responses, likes and comments about these photos. As emphasized in the article; capitalism, with its industry, information and information society, changes and transforms not only the communication, economy and social structure of the society but also the morality, education, manners, and norms of people and societies. Consequently, this kind of messages on social media are liked and the sender receives positive comments as in other examples.

(*continued on next page*)

Tab. 2: (continued)

Characteristics of Cynicism	Social Media Examples	Analysis
	("Youtube fenomenleri", 2018) People who are famous and earn money after forming a community on social media (phenomenon) are described. (Kızıltepe, 2018) Minister of Finance Naci Ağbal reveals that the government is going to get taxes from the persons, who earn financial income by promoting their products through social media accounts.	According to the news, the monthly earnings of famous social media celebrities are explained. According to the other URL, it is revealed that the celebrities will be taxed by the relevant ministry. Celebrities are able to receive advertisements and promote products through the pages they create on social media. Thus, they are able to direct the audience in line with their purposes.
Characteristics of Cynicism	**Social Media Examples**	**Analysis**
c) Goffman said, "a cynic performer can be emotionally aggressive by getting pleasure from something that the audience takes seriously".	(Zero TEK, 2017) It can be comprehended that a person is cynical about something the community takes seriously and s/he may be aggressive by getting a certain pleasure with this situation.	In the video s/he shared on social media, it can be observed that the person is cynical about a phenomenon that provides for the formation of beliefs, values, and norms of people and societies; and even as Goffman emphasizes, s/he can play as s/he wishes with something that social media viewers take very seriously and s/he is aggressive and happy about this.
	("Son dakika", 2018) On 11 March 2018, a plane crashed, and 11 women died, this is an example to it.	Both the media and the Prime Minister are forced to condemn the provoked social media attacks about the persons, who died while returning to Turkey after they went to Dubai for a bachelor party. It is also affirmed by thinkers and data miners that Twitter is the most effective social media tool in this regard. People may not care about the values of other people in the community they live in and the consequences of significant events (painful mother, father, spouse and child).

Tab. 2: (continued)

Characteristics of Cynicism	Social Media Examples	Analysis
d) A cynic actor can take an unprofessional pleasure from his/her deceptive behaviors and from his/her own deception.	("Russell Wilson eşinin", 2018) The news is about a couple of singers (woman) and American football (man) that share the photos of their bedrooms including the man's wife.	According to the news shared in digital media, a couple can disclose the scene of the bedroom, which is private for most people, through the social media to the whole world. The report also mentions that the person, who took the photo was very successful and received positive responses about the photos. The couple exhibits a behavior that is not accepted in most cultures and societies, and it is comprehended that the couple did this for getting pleasure and likes on social media.
	(Sosyal Göz, 2018) It explains a person, who is cynical, becomes a social celebrity by the cynical things s/he shares.	Celebrities on social media share cynical attitudes, speeches, postures and visuals in a totally cynical approach. The person, mentioned in "Sosyal Göz", has 7 million 136 thousand followers, and his/her film is watched by over 1 million people.
	(Çelik, 2018) On the other hand, in Hürriyet newspaper, a celebrity of social media is mentioned together with this person's films and high income.	In the other URL, it is declared that children are interacting with the videos they are watching, and they want to become Youtuber since they think social media is the only way to become famous. For both individuals and children; knowledge, wisdom and virtue are being replaced by being famous, getting likes and the factors that can be associated with the self of a person.
	In ("Enes Batur'un aylık", 2018) mentions that even children would like to become Youtuber and famous.	Also, they start to think that they can earn money when they are developing their selves and improve the social status.

(*continued on next page*)

Tab. 2: (continued)

Characteristics of Cynicism	Social Media Examples	Analysis
	("Rihanna'nın paylaşımı", 2018) It is disclosed that a famous singer has received many positive comments when s/he shares pictures without wearing lingerie.	Relevant news reveals the characteristics of the vision shared by the famous singer for contributing positively to his/her personal image. The report describes the body of the famous singer as well as the interesting clothes and accessories that surround her/his body. These photos of the famous singer are being largely admired by fans.
e) A cynic actor does not believe in the role s/he plays and is not fascinated by the role s/he plays.		
Jothimani, Bhadani & Shankar's (2015) research is an example of this statement.		

of the social structures and the people who form up the society are addressed with a cynical approach, the sarcasm is approached negatively, it is understood from the news that they even want to punish these persons themselves. On the other hand, according to Tab. 2, it is understood that the cynicism of Goffman, as mentioned in the article d), the persons do not approach negatively to sarcasm unless the intellectual, historical, religious, political actors, values and signs are addressed cynically. Yet, according to social and new media examples, the persons forming the society admire the sharings like this. The visual, conceptual and auditory images in the content of the actor in the article b) of Tab. 2, are whether accepted or not by today's society and social structures. According to Tab. 2, people, who want to be famous by sharing their naked photos and showing bodies and bedrooms, are appreciated by the audience. In addition, some people who want to be famous display cynical approaches, abnormal behaviors in digital, new and social media or they use a prominent phenomenon for the society, and they direct the audience that monitor the social media scene. In other words, some "cynical" sharing, classified in the behavioral examples in the article d) in Tab. 2 are affirmed by those who form the community. It is also comprehended from the social media examples that the celebrities exhibit their sharings and that the social media scene is used by brands for advertising since the audience watches. Finally, we understand that the celebrities earn an income through advertising. As observed in social media examples, people exhibit their self in the social media scene and have interactions that lead to the formation of the self. In fact, individuals are gaining new roles and status while nourishing their selves, and they can even earn their fame by adding new roles and statuses to their existing self, role and status, and even earn money through the fame.

Conclusion

As the philosophers referred to in the article emphasize, people are the actors in the system of social structure, thought and behavior. Moreover, the actors are active in the system of social structure, thoughts and behaviors; have roles and status. As people enter into interaction, share, participate, communicate and cooperate with society, social structures, technology and other people in their lives; they comply with, identify and internalize the systems of society, social structures, thoughts and behaviors. Thus, the person tends to conform to the behavior of family, work, group, community and society. Therefore, there are norms, laws, morality and values that the actor must obey. According to Goffman, people are actors in the scenes of life, and people show their performances on the stage formed by set, display window and decor. Goffman distinguishes between a "sincere" actor and a "cynical" actor. The sincere performer is one who is convinced that the impression of reality which he stages is the real reality, while the cynical performer is the otherwise. The approach of Goffman about the concept of "sincerity" is examined at Istanbul Aydın University in the doctoral dissertation called "Transformation of Personal and Brand Image Management in Social Media". By a dichotomy, Goffman describes the situations that are not "sincere" as the "cynical".

The philosophy of cynicism dates back to Ancient Greece and to Diogenes. According to the philosophy of cynicism and their representatives, the most prominent facts are freedom, self-sufficiency and free speech. According to the philosophy of cynicism, school and its representatives; the condemnation of Socrates condemnation to death and his execution is lawful but not fair. And therefore, cynics do not obey nor comply with norms, laws, morality and values established by social structure, thought and behavior systems, and do not identify themselves with them; and cynical person (actors) do not conform to the behaviors of family, work, group, community and society. Today, the thoughts and behaviors of cynic people can be described as guilty, insane and unhealthy. Foucault explains this situation with the creation of a great power tool in modern societies with the formation of norms and constraints by capitalism. According to him, thus, the individuals conform to the society and social structures with certain norms, moral values and constraints created by the power tool. On the other hand, according to Foucault, those who do not conform to the norms and constraints created by capitalism and power relations are defined as criminals, sick and mad people through society and social structures. In addition, according to him, the medicine, which is about isolating the normal from the abnormal, is also effectively used.

According to the organizational research referred to in the article, the actor's performance is measured by the "productivity production". According to consumeristic research, the actor's performance is the "consumption". Consequently, according to the relations of power, capitalism, organizational, marketing and brand management; actors (individuals) are expected to comply with the norms and laws created by the thought and behavior systems formed within the social system, to conform to them, even to identify themselves with them and perform their role (produce and consume) as the actors in a scene. Likewise, social media is a scene and people adopt the behavior of others in the social media scene; explain who they are and what characteristics they have within the framework of their knowledge, beliefs, and thoughts; and present themselves and receive comments of other on the stage they present themselves. Hence, they exhibit both existing identifies and selves while they want to achieve the ideal and desired identities and selves.

The cynicism, the philosophy of cynicism and the behaviors included in the concept of cynicism that are emphasized by Goffman are also expressed and exhibited in social media through daily life practices; as in the same historical context. As it is comprehended and explained with the social media examples in the article, although the actors are aware that their behaviors do not conform to the behaviors, norms, and rules of the society and they will be punished by law; they are "cynical" about the beliefs and values that the society owns and they do not care about the values and beliefs of the people that form the society and social structures. Moreover, the law and medical science do not accept such behaviors as observed in the examples. Persons in social media samples can direct the audience's beliefs to achieve other goals; therefore, they are considered unfair according to the law and they may lose their rights. On the other hand, in social media, people can receive positive reactions, likes and comments with their abnormal, cynical message. Instead of knowledge, wisdom and virtue; being liked and being famous become more popular for both children and individuals. Even, persons can earn money when they are developing themselves and raise their social status. Accordingly, the characteristics of Goffman's cynicism are realized in digital, new and social media that work with the digital code. As emphasized in the article, capitalism, with its industry, information and information society, changes and transforms not only the communication, economy and social structure of the society but also the morality, education, manners, proprieties and norms of individuals and societies.

On the other hand, concepts of cynicism in the history, digital cynicism do not mean sharing "cynical" conceptual, auditory and visual messages. Cynicism and digital cynicism signify virtue as they signified throughout the history. The concept of virtue includes the concepts of wisdom, courage, justice and moderation as the philosophers emphasize. Cynics advocate expressing truth, reality, liberation, free expression and they tell the truth; they protect their friends and bite their enemies for their friends. Moreover, they warn the people about *normal* persons to tend to conform to the social influence and carry out the daily duties and experiences, about the scene, to which they tend to conform. Snowden, who warned about the scene, can be guilty according to US law, even though he said truth and reality in honesty, as Socrates did. The concepts of cynicism and cynic philosophy, which date back to the Antiquity, are realized both in the internet, digital, new and social media environments that work with digital code, and cynics explain the negative effects of holistic structures formed by digital code on climate and technological convergence. This article suggests that there is a need to carry out a study on the hypothesis, "Hacktivists act like digital cynics", which is a subject that is investigated in social sciences.

Bibliography

Argon, T. ve Ekinci, S. (2016). İlk ve Ortaokul Öğretmenlerinin Örgütsel Özdeşleşme ve Örgütsel Sinizm Düzeylerine İlişkin Görüşleri. Abant İzzet Baysal Fakültesi Eğitim Fakültesi Dergisi, 16(1), 1–19.

Arkonaç, S. A. (2016). İnsan İnsan İçinde: Ana Akım ve Eleştirel Sosyal Psikoloji. İstanbul: Hiperlink Yayınları.

Arslan, A. (2017). İlkçağ Felsefe Tarihi: Sofistlerden Platon'a. İstanbul: İstanbul Bilgi Üniversitesi Yayınları.

Aytekin, E. (2018, March 2). Küresel güç mücadelesinin yeni aracı siber savaş. Anadolu Ajansı. Retrieved from https://aa.com.tr/tr/turkiye/kuresel-guc-mucadelesinin-yeni-araci-siber-savas/1077945 on 4 May 2018.

Baggini, J. (2013, Jul 10). In praise of cynicism. The Guardian. Retrieved from https://www.theguardian.com/world/2013/jul/10/in-praise-of-cynicism on 26 March 2018.

Barlas, H. C. (2017, November 14). Aleyna Tilki oyuncak penisli fotoğraf paylaştı! Sosyal medyayı salladı. Sözcü. Retrieved from http://www.sozcu.com.tr/hayatim/magazin-haberleri/aleyna-tilki-oyuncak-penisli-fotograf-paylasti-sosyal-medyayi-salladi/ on 15 April 2018.

Blog sözlük. (2017, April 18). Atatürk Heykelinin Üzerine Oturup Alay Eden Kadın [Video file]. Retrieved from https://www.youtube.com/watch?v=QvK3SawuQEs on 19 April 2018.

Bourse, M. & Yücel, H. (2012). İletişim Bilimlerinin Serüveni. İstanbul: Ayrıntı Yayınları.

Boush, D., Kim, C. H., Kahle, L. & Batra, R. (1993). Cynicism and Conformity as Correlates of Trust in Product Information Sources. Journal of Current Issues and Research in Advertising, 15, 71–79.

Candan, H. (2013). Örgütsel Sinizm ve İşgören Performansına Olası Etkileri. Kahramanmaraş Sütçü İmam Üniversitesi İktisadi ve İdari Bilimler Fakültesi Dergisi, 3(1), 181–194. Retrieved from http://iibfdergisi.ksu.edu.tr/issue/10266/125924 on 8 June 2018.

Cevizci, A. (2017). Büyük Felsefe Sözlüğü. İstanbul: Say Yayınları.

Cynics. (n.d.). Retrieved from The Internet Encyclopedia of Philosophy http://www.iep.utm.edu/cynics/ on 22 February 2018.

Çelik, E. (2018, May 4). Milyoner de olabilir, büyük zarar da görebilir: Eyvah çocuğum YouTuber oldu. Hürriyet. Retrieved from http://www.hurriyet.com.tr/yazarlar/ece-celik/milyoner-de-olabilir-buyuk-zarar-da-gorebilir-eyvah-cocugum-youtuber-oldu-40825434 on 6 May 2018.

Durkheim, E. (2012). Sosyoloji Dersleri (A. Berkay, Trans.). İstanbul: İletişim Yayınları.

Durkheim, E. (2014a). Toplumsal İşbölümü (Ö. Ozankaya, Trans.). İstanbul: Cem Yayınevi.

Durkheim, E. (2014b). Sosyolojik Yönetimin Kuralları (Ö. Doğan, Trans.). Ankara: Doğu Batı Yayınları.

Duverger, M. (2014). Toplum Bilimlerinde Araştırma Yöntem ve Teknikleri (Ö. Ozankaya, Trans.). İstanbul: Cem Yayınevi.

Enes Batur'un aylık kazancı şoke etti. (2018, May 2). CNNTürk.com. Retrieved from https://www.cnnturk.com/magazin/enes-baturun-aylik-kazanci-soke-etti?page=1on 6 May 2018.

Ertürk, Y. D. (2011). Sosyal Psikoloji Ders Notları. İstanbul: İstanbul Üniversitesi İletişim Fakültesi.

Ertürk, Y. D. (2017). Davranışlarımız ve Biz: Sosyal Psikoloji Bakışıyla Kalabalık İçinde Ben Olmak. İstanbul: Pozitif Yayınları.

Fama Haber. (2017, Jan 2). Barbaros Şansal'ın olay yaratan videosu [Video file]. Retrieved from https://www.youtube.com/watch?v=ZhFQEwzSKKY on 8 May 2018.

Foucault, M. (1995). Discipline and Punish: The Birth of the Prison (A. Sheridan, Trans.). New York: Vintage Books.

Foucault, M. (2008). The Goverment of Self and Others: Lectures at the College de France: 1982–1983 (A. Davidson,Trans.). Chippenham and

Eastbourne: Palgrave Macmillan, Printed and Bound in Great Britain by CPI Antony Rowe.

Foucault, M. (2015a). İktidarın Gözü, (İ. Ergüden, Trans.). İstanbul: Ayrıntı Yayınları.

Foucault, M. (2015b). Kelimeler ve Şeyler, İnsan Bilimlerinin Bir Arkeolojosi (M. A. Kılıçbay, Trans.). Ankara: İmge Kitabevi.

Foucault, M. (2015c). Öznenin Yorumbilgisi (F. Keskin, Trans.). İstanbul: İstanbul Bilgi Üniversitesi Yayınları.

Foucault, M. (2015d). Biyopolitikanın Doğuşu, (A. Tayla, Trans.). İstanbul: İstanbul Bilgi Üniversitesi Yayınları.

Foucault, M. (2015e). Büyük Kapatılma, (İ. Ergüden & F. Keskin, Trans.). İstanbul: Ayrıntı Yayınları.

Foucault, M. (2016). Özne ve İktidar, (İ. Ergüden & O. Akınhay, Trans.). İstanbul: Ayrıntı Yayınları.

Fuchs, C. (2016). Sosyal Medya: Eleştirel Bir Giriş (D. Saraçoğlu & İ. Kalaycı, Trans.). Ankara: NotaBene Yayınları.

Goffman, E. (1978). The Presentation of Self in Everyday Life. London: Penguin Books.

Goffman, E. (2014). Günlük Yaşamda Benliğin Sunumu (B. Cezar, Trans.). İstanbul: Metis Yayıncılık.

Güney, S. (2012). Sosyal Psikoloji. Ankara: Nobel Akademik Yayıncılık.

Güngör, N. (2013). İletişim Kuramlar ve Yaklaşımlar. Ankara: Ekinoks Yayın Dağıtım.

Güven, E. (2016). Tüketimde Sinik Tutum: Tüketici Sinizminin Sebep ve Sonuçları. İşletme Araştırmaları Dergisi, 8(2), 152–174. DOI:10.20491/isarder.2016.174.

Habermas, J. (1996). İletişimsel Eylem Kuramı, Eylem Rasyonelliği ve Toplumsal Rasyonelleşme, İşlevselci Aklın Eleştirisi Üzerine (M. Tüzel, Trans.). İstanbul: Kabalcı Yayınevi.

İnceoğlu, M. (2011). Tutum, Algı, İletişim. Ankara: Ekinoks Yayın Dağıtım.

Jothimani, D., Bhadani, A, K. & Shankar, R. (2015). Towards Understanding the Cyncisim of Social Networking Sites: An Operations Management Perspective, Procedia - Social and Behavioral Sciences, 189, 117–132.

Kağıtçıbaşı, Ç. & Cemalcılar, Z. (2015). Dünden Bugüne İnsan ve İnsanlar, Sosyal Psikolojiye Giriş. İstanbul: Evrim Yayınevi.

Kalaycı, N. (2015). Bir Parrhesiastes Olarak Diogenes. In H. Tepe & B. Çotuksöken (Eds.), Sinoplu Filozof Diogenes: Anadolu'da Felsefeye Yolculuk (pp. 73–89) II. Ankara: Türkiye Felsefe Kurumu.

Kaplan, A, M. & Hanlein, M. (2010). Users of The World, Unite! The Challenges and Oppurtunities of Social Media. Business Horizons, 53(1), 59–68. DOI:10.1016/j.bushor.2009.09.003.

Karacaoğlu, K. & İnce, F. (2012). Brandes, Dharwadker ve Dean'in (1999) Örgütsel Sinizm Ölçeği Türkçe Formunun Geçerlilik ve Güvenilirlik Çalışması: Kayseri Organize Sanayi Bölgesi Örneği. Business and Economics Research Journal, 3(3), 77–92.

Kart, M. E. (2015). Örgütsel Sinizm: Bağlamsal Performans ve Etik İdeoloji. Ankara: Nobel Akademi Yayıncılık.

Kızıltepe, O. (2018, April 11). Sosyal Medyadan Reklam Yapıp Para Kazanan Fenomenlere Vergi Zorunluluğu Geliyor. Haberler.com. Retrieved from https://www.haberler.com/sosyal-medyadan-reklam-yapip-para-kazanan-10744721-haberi/ 19 April 2018.

Kutsal, S. (2017, August 3). Wikileaks: Mikrofon ve kameraların kontrolü CIA'de!. Digitalage. Retrieved from http://digitalage.com.tr/wikileaks-mikrofon-ve-kameralarin-kontrolu-ciade/ on 12 May 2018.

Laertios, D. (2017). Ünlü Filozofların Yaşamları ve Öğretileri (C. Şentuna, Trans.). İstanbul: Yapı Kredi Yayınları.

Luck, G. (2011). Köpeklerin Bilgeliği: Antikçağ Kiniklerinden Metinler (O. Özügül, Trans.). İstanbul: Say Yayınları.

Mattelart, A. (2004). Bilgi Toplumunun Tarihi (H. Y. Altınel, Trans.). İstanbul: İletişim Yayınları.

McLuhan, M. & Powers, B. R. (1992). The Global Village. US: Oxford University Press.

Mead, G. H. (2017). Zihin, Benlik ve Toplum (Y. Erdem, Trans.). Ankara: Heretik Basın Yayın.

Odou, P. & Pechpeyrou, P. (2011). Consumer Cynicisim: From Resistance to Anti-Consumption in a Disenchanted World? European Journal of Marketing, 45(11/12), 1799–1808.

Parsons, T. (1968). Toplumsal Eylemin Yapısı, (A. Bölükbaşı, Trans.). Sakarya: Sakarya Üniversitesi Kültür Yayınları.

Paylaşımlarıyla tepki çeken öğretmen meslekten ihraç edildi. (2018, March 9). Milliyet. Retrieved from http://www.milliyet.com.tr/gundem/paylasimlariyla-tepki-ceken-ogretmen-meslekten-ihrac-edildi-2624510 on 19 April 2018.

Platon. (2014). Sokrates'in Savunması. İstanbul: Everest Yayınları.

Rihanna'nın paylaşımı yine çok konuşuldu. (2018, April 16). Turktime.com. Retrieved from http://www.turktime.com/haber/rihanna-nin-paylasimi-yine-cok-konusuldu/465373 on 19 April 2018.

Russell Wilson eşinin seksi fotoğraflarını çekti! (2018, Jan 4). Medyafaresi. Retrieved from http://www.medyafaresi.com/foto-galeri/russell-wilson-esinin-seksi-fotograflarini-cekti/853693/2 on 20 April 2018.

Son dakika: Türk özel jeti İran'da düştü. (2018, March 11). Hürriyet. Retrieved from http://www.hurriyet.com.tr/gundem/son-dakika-turk-ozel-jeti-iranda-dustu-ucakta-bulunan-11-kisi-oldu-40768590 on 20 March 2018.

Sosyal Göz. (2018, March 20). Kerimcan Durmaz, Samet Liçina, Selin Ciğerci Dubai de Şahin Yanlıyo Ayol [Video file]. Retrieved from https://www.youtube.com/watch?v=oamdQxyK95c on 22 March 2018.

Sosyal medyanın en çok konuşulan çıplak fotoğrafları. (2017, October 9). Hürriyet. Retrieved from http://www.hurriyet.com.tr/galeri-sosyal-medyanin-en-konusulan-ciplak-fotograflari-40604246?p=2 on 9 April 2018.

Şimşek, S. (2015). Polisliğin Kronik Hastalığı. Hitit Üniversitesi Sosyal Bilimler Enstitüsü Dergisi, 8(1), 253–271.

T24. (2018). Edward Snowden: Cambridge Analytica skandalında Facebook kurban değil, suç ortağı. Retrieved from http://t24.com.tr/haber/edward-snowden-cambridge-analytica-skandalinda-facebook-kurban-degil-suc-ortagi,586534 on 20 March 2018.

Tan, H. (2017a). Pazarlama Amaçlı Halkla İlişkilerin Sosyal Medyadaki Uygulamalarını Starbucks Markası Üzerinden İncelemek. 2. Genç Bilim İnsanları Sempozyumu. İstanbul: İstanbul Aydın Üniversitesi Yayınları, 119–135.

Tan, H. (2017b). To Examine Reasons of Social Media Usage Through Personal and Brand Image Management. In Ö. Çankaya, H. Yengin & D. Yengin (Eds.), Communication and Technology Congress-CTC 2017.Proceedings of the 1st CTC of İstanbul Aydin University New Media Department (pp. 105–115). İstabul, Turkey. Doi: 10.7456/ctc_2017_08.

Tasner, M. (2011). Anında Pazarlama, Web 3.0 Pazarlama Kılavuzu (A. Özer, Trans.). İstanbul: MediaCat Kitapları.

Timuçin, A. (2004). Felsefe Sözlüğü. İstanbul: Bulut Yayınları.

Ulus, Ç. (2017, June 30). 'Blogger' anneye çocuk istismarı suçlaması! GazeteVatan. Retrieved from http://www.gazetevatan.com/-blogger-anneye-cocuk-istismari-suclamasi--1080670-gundem/ on 19 April 2018.

Üçok, D. and Torun, A. (2014). Tükenmişliği Etkileyen Olumsuz Tutum ve Beklentiler: Sinik Tutum ve Psikolojik Sözleşme İhlali Algısı Üzerine Bir

Araştırma. Atatürk Üniversitesi İktisadi ve İdari Bilimler Dergisi, 28(1), 231–250.

Vanderstraeten, R. (2012). Talcott Parsons and the Enigma of Secularization. European Journal of Social Theory, 16(1), 69–84.

Wallace, R. A. & Wolf, A. (2015). Çağdaş Sosyoloji Kuramları: Klasik Geleneğin Gelişmesi, (L. Elburuz, & M. R. Ayas, Trans.). Ankara: Doğu Batı Yayınlar.

We Are Social. (2018, Jan 29). Digital in 2018. Slideshare. Retrieved from www.slideshare.net/wearesocial/digital-in-2018-global-overview-86860338 on 15 March 2018.

Weber, M. (2012a). Ekonomi ve Toplum: Cilt-1 (L. Boyacı, Trans.). İstanbul: Yarın Yayınları.

Weber, M. (2012b). Ekonomi ve Toplum: Cilt-2, (L. Boyacı, Trans.). İstanbul: Yarın Yayınları.

Weber, M. (2013). Protestan Ahlakı ve Kapitalizm Ruhu (G. Rızaoğlu, Trans.). İstanbul: Oda Yayınları.

Yalçınkaya, A. (2014). Türkiye'de Örgütsel Sinizm: 2007–2012 Yılları Arasındaki Çalışmalar Üzerine Bir Değerlendirme. İşgüç Endüstri İlişkileri ve İnsan Kaynakları Dergisi, 16(3), 106–130.

Yavaşgel, E. (2014). İletişimin Sosyo-Politiği. İstanbul: Der Kitabevi.

Youtube fenomenleri ne kadar kazanıyor? (2018, Dec 5). CNNTürk. Retrived from https://www.cnnturk.com/ekonomi/youtube-fenomenleri-ne-kadar-kazaniyor on 20 December 2018.

Zero TEK. (2017, July 2). İslam ile dalga geçen kadın [Video file]. Retrieved from https://www.youtube.com/watch?v=X5W5QDnlDTs&has_verified=1 26 March 2018.

Tamer Bayrak and And Algül

Effects of Frame Rate in Virtual Reality

Abstract: The new media technologies offer the virtual communication environment which is the digital copy of the real world for individuals. In the virtual environment, the factor of presence is one of the critical components required for an effective virtual environment. An increase in the sense of presence facilitates user's participation and interaction or, in other words, user's immersion in virtual reality. This chapter examines the effects of the frame rate factor – an important element in the formation of the presence – on the users of Virtual Reality (VR). Some of the effects induced by the use of the VR are associated with the features of the provided virtual environment. One of these features is the frame rate. It was studied in the research whether Frame per Second (FPS) change had any effects on the users during the use of head mounted displays or not, and if so, what these effects were. Through a suitable sampling with 50 people, the users experienced four different VR games with various levels of FPS change; users' performance was observed during the game and at the end of the game; and they were asked questions in order to measure their experiences of use. The result of the research is that the FPS change in the game caused users to give physical and verbal reactions in the games played by wearing a virtual reality headset. The strong FPS change increases immersion and hence enhances the sense of presence. While this increases the physical reactions of users, it also enables them to get pleasure from the game and enjoy it. In this sense, it is possible to state that the FPS change enhances users' enjoyment. Nevertheless, it turned out that the FPS change led to use-induced negative symptoms and multiplied the negative symptoms.

Keywords: frame rate, FPS, virtual reality, virtual environment, presence

Introduction

People who struggle to develop communication, to shorten the process of its realization, and to have various channels in this sense lead to the rapid transformation of the new media. The communication tools which were called the conventional media, and which adopted a one-way communication model, began to meet users under the name "new media technologies" upon the origination of the computer technology. Having included artificial intelligence and digital media into their scope, the new media carried communication to different dimensions by incorporating the Internet technology into their structure too. Virtual reality, which originated after the integration of the phenomenon of communication with the new media, is striking as the first product of this transformation.

Communication, an important requirement for people, maintains its existence within a continuous development by integrating with the technique acquired by people. As being the exchange of processed knowledge among individuals, communication satisfies the need of people for socialization. As stated by Van Dijk, the movement of processed knowledge among individuals commences with the processing of "bits" – the smallest building blocks of knowledge – with information (Van Dijk, 2016). Bits, which mean the meaningless pieces of data existing in a medium, are processed, and come together, with the knowledge that has occurred by previously completing this process and make up meaningful data sets. Having completed its transformation as a result of the processing of information, knowledge is used by the individual waiting to use it in order to complete the formation of new knowledge. Thanks to this, the knowledge formation cycle maintains its continuity.

The merging of the phenomenon of communication with the virtual reality technology became possible through the continuous development of the technique – the knowledge of producing. When human beings, who had tried to confine the technique – previously implemented in certain narrow and limited areas – throughout history, met the complex of techniques basically such as production techniques, techniques of warfare and hunting, and consumption techniques (e.g. clothes & finery and houses), they integrated with the technique that covered their whole life and that seemed like representing a quite important area to modern human beings (Ellul, 2003: 76).

The communication process in the new media is completed with the process of bit, data, and information, as Van Dijk stated in his work "The Network Society" (Van Dijk, 2016). According to this diagram, which represents a communication process resembling those of all other media, communication takes place at a profoundly rapid pace in terms of quality and quantity. A bit, the smallest unit of knowledge, is represented with 0 and 1 in the virtual environment. The bit sets that come together to form a meaningful whole make up data – quantifiable knowledge. The data which interact with the exogenous processed knowledge generate information, whereas information generates the processed knowledge (Yengin, 2014: 32). Fig. 1, represents the infinite cycle of the communication process between the source and the target in the new media, and the conventional communication processes also display major analogies. Presented by people so as to develop communication – a vital requirement of theirs – and the knowledge formation process – the requirement of communication, the virtual reality technology qualifies as an extension of all the new media technologies presented.

The new media technology provided the origination of communication media with complex digital systems. One of the most important elements of

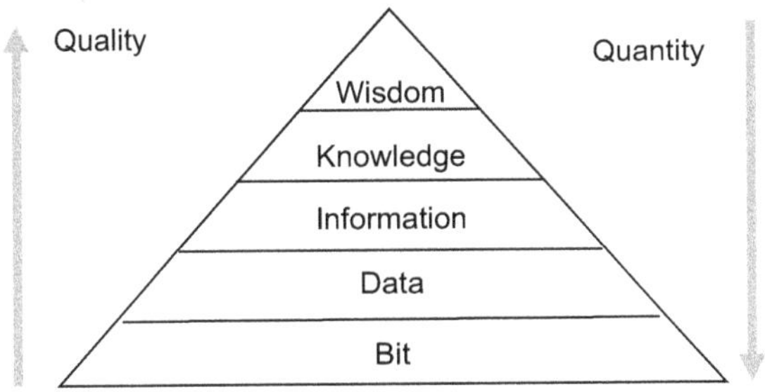

Fig. 1: The Pyramid of Information Processing (Van Dijk, 2016).

these media is the virtual reality technology. While the virtual reality technology isolates the user from the real world, it enables the user to be positioned in the virtual environments that have been designed digitally, that are copies of reality, and that have unique features. An individual who has a chance of possessing a new identity (virtual identity) in these media is able to carry out the actions he/she cannot express in real life. With this technology, which requires robust computer hardware, Internet providing tools, and virtual reality technology tools, the individual experiences some adverse symptoms as a result of the intensive information provided by technology. The symptoms, one of the most serious obstacles to the dissemination of this technology, constitute an essential factor to understand the effects of virtual reality on an individual. In this sense, it becomes important to examine the frame rate, which has a quite significant share in the development of the virtual reality technology as well as in the occurrence of symptoms as a result of use, as a research subject. The frame rate increases during the acceleration of the image but decreases during its deceleration. Making up the content of the study and having a quite determining role in the virtual reality technology, the frame rate was not further quantified, and the information provided by PlayStation was taken as the basis.

Virtual Reality in Communication Studies

Communication maintains its existence as a quite important need of humanity. In this sense, the phenomenon of communication, whose importance has never diminished throughout history, proves that a human being is a social being. Communication is the fundamental condition for producing the social life and for coexistence. Any meaning produced in the communication relationship is produced socially and only realized in the context of the production relationships formed with other people (Yaylagül, 2016: 14). All thinkers who have dealt with the problems in the field of communication from McLuhan to Ong and Innis agree that the media, whereby people communicate with each other, affect their ways of thinking and consequently the society they live in either directly or indirectly (Ong, 1995; McLuhan, 2001; Innis, 2006).

Derived from the Latin word "communis," communication has made the transformation of the conventional media into the new media unavoidable as the process of sending, receiving, processing, re-sending, re-receiving, re-processing, etc. of meaning-loaded symbols performed between an individual and another individual (or other individuals) (Oskay, 1993: 309–310). An individual's desire to develop the communication channels he/she acquired through the conventional media and his/her endless demands resulted in the replacement of the one-way communication model by the two-way communication model (Karadağ, 2017: 724). An individual who became both a consumer and a producer upon the origination of computer and Internet technologies demanded the new media technologies as well and provided the acceleration of globalization through the increasing of the diversity of channels of communication.

The new media technologies offer the virtual communication environment – the digital copy of the real world – for individuals. Visualization is the most characteristic feature in the virtual environment that provides an individual with an opportunity for creating a new identity. Due to visualization, which underlies the phenomenon of communication in the virtual environment, virtual reality refers to the expansion of the views of the real world. This expansion intends to compensate for the shrinkage of distances resulting from the time compression created by instantaneous telecommunications (Virilio, 2003: 18–19). With the virtual identity an individual has created, he/she sort of purifies himself/herself by displaying the behavior that he/she cannot display in his/her real life in this virtual environment, where the duration of completion of communication is shortened. For a human being, entertainment further enhances the submissiveness whereby he/she wants to forget himself/herself in the entertainment (Adorno, 2012: 75). Therefore, an individual is further wedded to the new media technologies, in which his/her submissiveness increases, by experiencing "catharsis" in the virtual environment, in which a techno-copy of everything is available.

The virtual reality technology is based on the simulation of the real world. In the virtual environment, where the codes composed digitally of 0 and 1 come together and make up meaningful entirety, reality now leaves its place to "simulacra," which have replaced reality. Frequently mentioned by Baudrillard, simulacra digitally occupy a space in the virtual environment, have an individual feel as if they were real, and paralyze the individual's perception of reality (Baudrillard, 2005). An individual who has been affected by what he/she has seen becomes completely open to the manipulations by the section that has produced the content. The virtual reality technology, which has now become a commodity for the user who has adopted the technological tool he/she uses as the hope for purifying himself/herself, begins to encourage consumption, as all other objects of production do. A commodity whose single use-value is its exchange-value, and which is in the position of an object of mass production makes the consumer passive, makes him/her indifferent to politics, and objectifies him/her (Hitchcock, 2013: 76). When considered from this perspective, the section that produces content for the virtual reality technology works to increase the pleasure obtained from the environment, while consumers encourage production by consuming the products at a profoundly rapid pace. In order for the virtual reality environment content to be produced, it should be subject to consumption and this consumption should be continuous, as in all other media environments. Thus, user's enjoyment is acknowledged as essential.

Virtual Reality Studies

Virtual reality is used within the scope of various practices from entertainment to product development as well as from psychological treatment methods to augmented reality studies – an extension of the virtual reality in various fields of education (Ottosson, 2002; Chen et al., 2015; Valmaggia et al., 2016; Freeman et al., 2017). Various purposeful or coincidental positive and negative results during and after the participation in the virtual reality environment are studied by researchers (Nichols et al., 2000a). Successful virtual reality should have qualities which mostly enhance the sense of presence in a virtual setting. This can be attained through generating the visual and sound contents in the virtual environment with the most realistic and unique features.

The senses of immersion and presence in the virtual reality environment occur as important concepts. In this context, the increase in users' senses of immersion and presence in the virtual reality environment and their interaction are acknowledged as important and it is seen that virtual reality studies are developed for an increase in this interaction. Accordingly, within the scope of virtual reality, the concept of immersion refers to the experience embracing an environment, as in an elevator, whereas enjoyment is defined as the sense of enjoyment or satisfaction during the virtual reality experience (Lin et al., 2002: 165). In virtual reality, presence is expressed as the sense of presence in the environment in which participants forget the real world and which arouses the sense that it is a place that they visit rather than a place that they see (Nichols et al., 2000a: 489).

The factor of presence is one of the critical components required for an effective virtual environment. An increase in the sense of presence facilitates user's participation and interaction or, in other words, user's immersion in virtual reality. The increase in the user's sense of presence depends on the fact that the virtual reality environment has features closest to reality as well as on its ability to reflect its unique features in the best way. However, unfavorable side effects which may negatively affect the next participation of a participant in the environment and overshadow its benefit may occur as side effects of presence in virtual reality. These side effects are defined with various designations as motion sickness and simulator sickness (McCauley and Sharkey, 1992: 313; Kolasinski, 1995: 2). It is also seen that the use-induced sicknesses are defined differently, namely "virtual reality-induced symptoms and effects" or "synthetic experience" (Cobb et al., 1999; Nichols et al.,2000b; Sharples et al., 2008).

It is stated that the factors which impair pictorial realism like the delay of visual feedback decrease the sense of presence, whereas reality and interaction increase the sense of presence (Welch et al., 1996: 263). Furthermore, it is explicit that a display medium or an image also has positive or negative effects on the sense of presence.

What kinds of effects wide and narrow fields of vision have in virtual reality is one of the investigated issues. Although it is stated that the field of vision and screen resolution affect the use of the virtual reality environment and cause motion sickness, it is expressed that they are not considered important factors which will cause visual stress by affecting user's physical activities and reactions (Stanney and Salvendy, 1998: 142). It is mentioned that users can develop more spatial awareness and a higher sense of presence with a greater field of vision (Usoh et al., 2000). Nevertheless, it is also expressed that users display more postural discomfort in the virtual reality environment due to the increase in the field of vision (Duh et al., 2001).

In their research, Lin et al. draw attention to the conclusion that presence, enjoyment and simulator sickness change as a function of the field of vision in the virtual reality environment (Lin et al., 2002: 164). They discovered that presence and simulator sickness increased depending on the increase in the field of vision and that there was, therefore, a positive correlation between presence and the sickness, whereas there was a negative correlation between enjoyment and the sickness. This demonstrates that there is a relationship among the field of vision, enjoyment of an image, and physical reactions (these reactions are predominantly the efforts of staying in balance while experiencing).

While another study reveals the complex relationships among presence, enjoyment, simulator sickness, and user interaction in the virtual reality environment (Lin and Parker, 2007: 423); Nichols et al. studied the relationship among presence, enjoyment, and simulator sickness and stated that there was no relationship between simulator sickness and enjoyment (Nichols et al., 2000a: 489).

It is suggested that ease of interaction, user's control over his/her actions, pictorial realism, duration of exposure to virtual reality, factors of social existence created by the presence of virtual actors and technological systemic factors in virtual reality are among the factors which affect the sense of presence (Stanley and Salvendy, 1998: 162).

Vision in a virtual environment is related to the features of the image displayed to the user. One of these features is the frame rate of an image. The concept is the refresh rate or the simulation rate or the rate at which the frames following the scene in motion are created (Pausch et al., 1992).

Users of the virtual reality technology perceive the images they see with this technology as if they were real. Perception of the virtual images produced as copies of reality as if they were real by the human brain depends on a high frame rate (the frequency of succession of images). Thanks to the feature which is a kind of a defect of the human eye and which provides the existence of conventional media tools like cinema, the dull images seen on the screen or the movie screen are displayed in rapid succession and the stable images leaving a mark on the eye by means of light are perceived as if they were in motion by the brain. In this regard, the perception of reality by the human brain increases to the extent of the increase in this projection rate, which also makes use of the dark environment. However, on the one hand, an increase in the frame rate gives rise to an increase in the perception of reality in the brain, but on the other, it leads to the triggering of some negative use-induced symptoms. Within this scope, the study aims to reveal whether the FPS change in the game has any effect on users depending on users' experiencing in the context of the uses and effects approach and, if yes, what kinds of effects FPS has. In the research section of the study, the users who participated voluntarily were made to play four high-resolution games called Eagle Flight, Robots Rescue, Driveclub, and Until Dawn (with slow and intensive FPS changes) and the experiences of the users during the games were observed. In this way, it was intended to determine the effects of the frame rate – a quite important and technical subject for the virtual reality technology – on users within the scope of the uses and effects approach.

Frame Rate in Virtual Reality

The virtual reality technology, whereby the phenomenon of communication has transformed and assumed a new form, is an extension of the computer and Internet technology. The requirement of a technology for another technology in order to be able to exist (Manovich, 2001: 30–40) is also the reason why the virtual reality technology cannot exist without the computer and Internet technology. The way in which technical knowledge forced technology to transform culminated in the fact that human beings found themselves in a new communication environment. In this sense, the virtual reality technology stands out as a software and hardware technology (King, 2016: 218) provided by the advanced computer technology. In this technology, where a techno-copy of real life is produced, the user joins a fully participated environment by wearing the headset placed into a helmet wearable to the head. The individual, whose relationship with the real environment is broken off completely, organizes his/her perception of reality entirely according to the virtual environment in the fully participated environment he/she has joined. Interacting with virtual objects, thanks to the technical equipment developed, the individual tries to adjust to the environment by adapting himself/herself according to the purpose of the encoding of the objects (Oppenheim, 1993: 215–217).

Virtual reality headsets, which are useful to get out of what is real and make a transition to the virtual world (Sherman and Craig, 2003: 135), are produced to work compatibly with computer hardware, an optical sensor, and controlling devices. A user who has worn the headset passes into the sensing field of the optical sensor and is positioned in the virtual environment designed for the device. Furthermore, the interaction of the individual also increases according to the content and quality of the image that comes to the eye of the user from the computer. To enhance the interaction, it is important to provide the consumer with the content produced for the virtual reality technology by means of the screens that will support a high frame rate (Sherman et al., 2009).

The frame rate is also defined as the number of frames per second (So et al., 2001). Moreover, the frame rate is also called the refresh rate by some authors. It shows how often the image buffer is examined and reflected in the screen (Barrett, 2004: 19). Used to mean the frame transferred to the screen per second, the frame rate determines the effect that a computer game leaves on the user. The frame rate, which is as important as sound, content, and image for a digital game, and the number of Frames per Second (FPS), which is the unit that quantifies the processor, ram, and video card performances of a computer, are

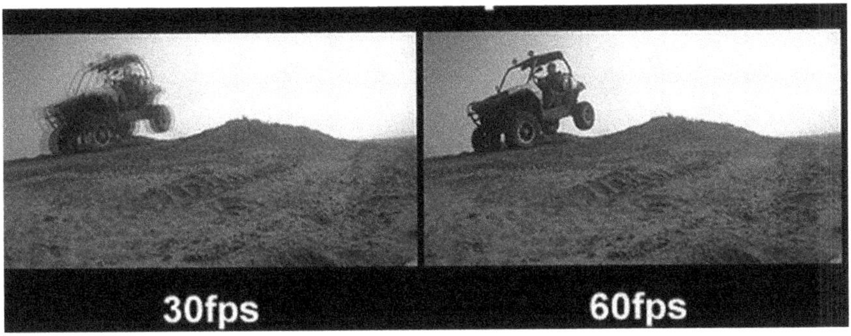

Image 1: The Visual Difference Between 30FPS and 60FPS (iWazzuu, 2010).

used as synonyms. When considered from this perspective, an image captured per second and with a frame number of 30FPS according to the graphic feature means an image in which 30 frames have been captured per second. Thus, the higher the FPS value in an image, the greater the motion sharpness of an image (Sherman and Craig, 2003: 135).

The FPS value in digital games varies according to the quality of the computer hardware. Nevertheless, the lowest FPS is 25, as seen in today's digital game sector. Given the present computer technology, this value indicates the level at which some standard computer hardware can run a game program. However, when the digital game platforms like Steam are considered, it is seen that the games offered for consumers are generally comprised of the games at the levels that will not disturb a player like 30FPS. This is because of the occurrence of freezing images, image persistence, and interrupted images when the value of 25FPS drops and because the FPS value is quite variable. The share of 5FPS in between prevents the player from experiencing these problems. However, since the amount of processed knowledge in the visual data increases with an increase in the FPS value, the program size also increases directly proportionally.

The compatibility of a digital game with the computer hardware determines the FPS value, whereas the perception capacity of the human eye determines the limits of this value. Additionally, the capacity of a human being to perceive the FPS value varies by individual. Therefore, it is rather difficult to answer the question "How many FPS can a human eye see?". One should look at the softness of the motion in order to give a meaning to the FPS that the human eye can perceive after a certain level. As the difference in the transition from one frame

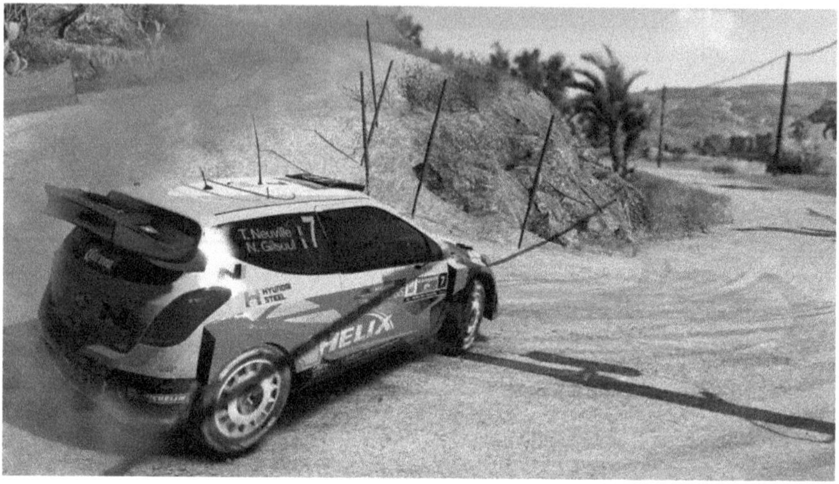

Image 2: Image Content at Lower than 30FPS (PlayStation.Store, 2015).

to another will be minor in an image with uncertain limits and sharpness (e.g., a foggy, rainy or cloudy image) due to the slow rate of motion and the great softness of the transition, the FPS value will not be important.

As a fast-moving object in front of the human eye blurs, it is perceived as if it was becoming fluent. For instance, a fast-moving car in an image of a car pass recorded by a stable video camera is transmitted to viewers in line with the technical adequacy of the video camera. When an image recorded by a video camera that does not support a high frame rate is paused, a blurry vehicle image is obtained. This image has an effect on the viewer as if the vehicle was fast. Nevertheless, this confines the reality of the image in the form of a message conveyed by means of a communication tool and negatively affects an individual's perception of reality.

A motion picture is known to play at 24FPS. However, when the image begins to decrease below 18FPS in an active movie, disturbing freezing and interrupted images begin to form in the images. Furthermore, a similar disturbing situation also occurs in the movies with an FPS value higher than 50FPS and with resolution of good quality. When the image starts to rise from this level, it sharpens and an individual who decodes the image with clear details begins to feel tired after a while or negative symptoms occur in the individual. In this sense, in order for a person to watch a movie without being disturbed, it is adequate for an image to be between 18 and 50FPS.

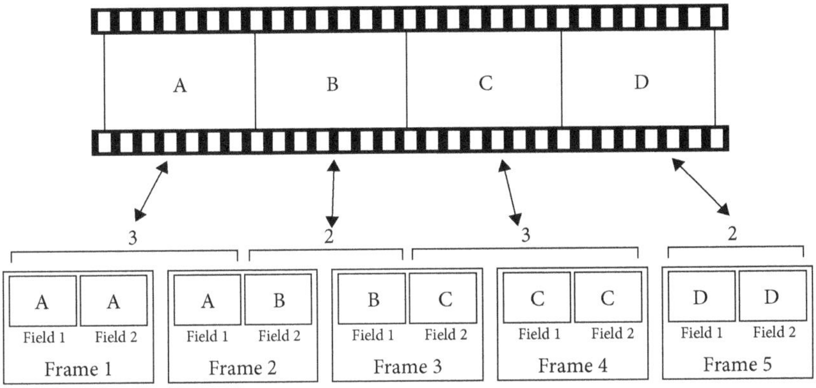

Fig. 2: The Cinematic Frame Rate (Motion compensated, n.d.).

The limits of the human eye and of computer hardware also reveal the importance of the harmony between light and darkness in an image (Pimentel and Teixeira, 1993). The difference in brightness between light and darkness causes one to perceive this difference easily. Hence, a human being sees a dark image that even occurs for a period of one-sixtieth of a second. For instance, since a black image provided in one-twenty-fourth of a second in a motion picture can be seen and perceived more clearly, a black image is provided at short intervals after each video frame at the cinema. Each movie frame is displayed three times one after another; the third frame is the transitional frame; and the following one frame is made black, thereby providing the transition between two actions. In this sense, the image is black for a very short period of time between the two actions. A movie watched at 24FPS in the technical sense is watched at 72FPS with this factor, whereby the refresh rate in the image is tripled; nevertheless, this does not disturb viewers. This is owing to the failure of the human eye to notice the dark images at this rate due to the structure of the human eye. Although a viewer who focuses considerably can notice black dots or interrupted images from time to time, it is impossible for a viewer to watch the whole movie with great attention; however, this does not constitute any obstacle to watching a movie.

The cinematic frame rate, which forms the basis for the logic of the frame rate in an image provided by the computer technology, was essentially discovered and used in the context of the limitations of the human eye so as to solve the problem of continuity. The frame rate of 24FPS was considerably increased with the frame rate that entered a different phase upon the origination of the conventional media tools. For instance, the perception of reality was considerably

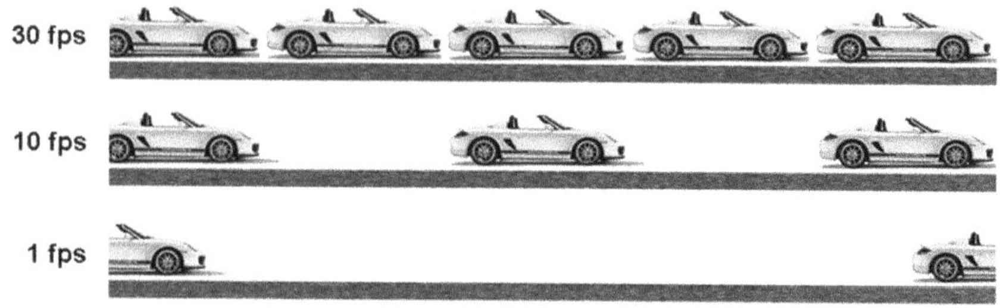

Image 3: Differences in Image Refresh Rates among FPS Values ("What is an action camera?", 2018).

strengthened with the black image that was reduced to as low as 1/100 of a second in a television operating at 100Hz frequency. In this sense, it is seen that light suppresses darkness and that the viewer can watch the image easily by not being able to perceive darkness.

Of the new media technologies that originated after the conventional media, the virtual reality technology has superior display features with frame rates greater than 60FPS. The frequency of dark images used to ensure continuity in a broadcast image in the conventional media tools has increased to high levels in virtual reality and, also with the inclusion of the 360 degrees image, an individual's perception of reality has quite increased. In this sense, full participation of an individual is ensured upon the increase in the number of frames captured per second (Yengin and Bayrak, 2018: 104–105) and the individual is exposed to use-induced negative symptoms. The basic reason for this is the inability of the body to react at the same level at which the brain reacts to the nearly real image seen by an individual. For instance, an individual in the simulation of a fast-moving car only experiences reality in the iconic sense. Due to such factors as the lack of movement, and of gravitational (the g-force) force, in the seat on which he/she sits, the individual is unable to support his/her perception of reality with his/her body; hence, the body is unable to keep up with the reactions of the brain to virtual objects in a nonreactive environment. The problem concerned is relatively solved through the production of reacting seats, treadmills, and wearable clothes fitted with sensors that simulate the factors required by the virtual environment. When considered from this perspective, it is seen that the frequency of the frame rate entirely affects the perception of reality in virtual reality and that technical tools to respond to physical reactions should inevitably be developed with this technology (Chayko, 2018: 211). Otherwise, the use of this technology by masses of people will remain limited.

A user interacts with the digital medium he/she is in according to the frequency of the number of frames captured per second and some defects in the human eye. These defects are necessary for the eye to detect the movement of the image during the frame frequency. For instance, the human eye in a dark environment can easily see the light instantly flashing on and off. A human being can detect and perceive the bright images on the screen that is continually flashing on and off during the frame rate. The defect in the eye comes into play at this very moment. The defect which enables the brain to process even the bright image that appears for a period of 1/200 of a second in a dark environment is defined as an afterimage.

This defect, which makes the existence of conventional media tools like cinema and of the subsequent new media tools possible, is the perception of the light coming to the human eye as if it was still in front of the eye despite the disappearance of its source. The receptors of the human eye are stimulated against sudden changes and then cannot return to their former state immediately. In this case, the brain goes on functioning in order to be able to process and it combines and processes the fragmentarily flashing image by using this defect of the eye.

The FPS sensitivity values of the human eye vary. In this sense, an image should have a value between 60FPS and 120FPS in order for the eye, which sees at values between 18FPS and 25FPS under normal conditions, to perceive the image on the digital screen as real. An image with such a value misleads the brain and can persuade it that the image does not indeed consist only of some digital content but is a real image. Nevertheless, headaches occur since the processing capacity of the brain increases when the FPS value increases in an image. With the inability of the body to support the brain, some negative symptoms begin to occur and this reaches the extent that will require ending the use of the device.

The problems experienced in the use of the virtual reality technology are related to both the high frame rate and the ability or inability of a human being to see, i.e. the fields which remain out of his/her control. A human being, who is a social being, prefers those fields which he/she can see and rule when building his/her living space. Trying to eliminate all elements which pose a threat to his/her life, a person continues his/her life by forming a community with the individuals who think like him/her. This inevitably led to the occurrence of those mechanisms which provided harmony and coexistence in social relations. Theorized by Foucault (2003) and formed by Orwell (2016), the panoptic society understanding refers to the utopia of a society which is caused by the occurring mechanisms and in which people are continually being spied on. In this respect, by nature, a human being is afraid of what he/she cannot see and rule or what he/she sees but cannot give any meaning to and worries about the fields remaining

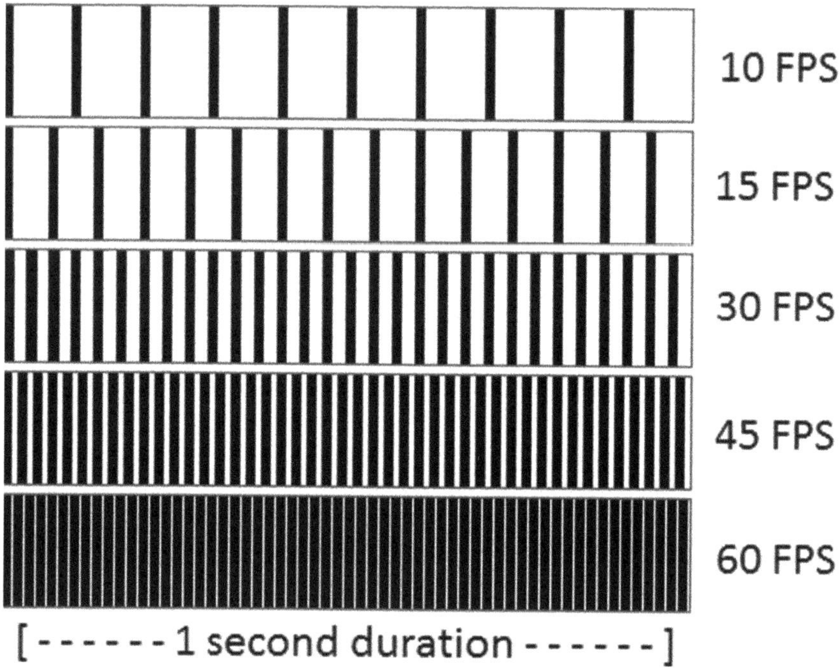

Fig. 3: The Differences in Image Frequency among the FPS Values (Staff; 2014).

out of his/her field of vision in a panoptic social order. A person who does not want to become disconnected from the daily flow of information in the panoptic social order, which has further been clarified, thanks to the electronic networks that have entirely surrounded the world, worries at the moment when he/she feels inadequacy in the information he/she has obtained from what he/she has seen or heard. In the virtual reality environment as well, the ability of users to perceive the environment and to see the images in the environment clearly is important for them to adapt to the environment. Hence, the FPS changes created in the virtual reality technology that is currently in use in order for users to experience more fun and pleasure bring about serious obstacles that restrict the ability of users to see and hear as well as their mobility. In this sense, the negative symptoms occurring in users depending on the FPS change were investigated in the context of the uses and effects approach. For this purpose, the users were made to play the four games mentioned below and the effects on the individuals were examined.

The game requirements for the four games used within the scope of the research are as follows:

The game "Eagle Flight" is played by one player. The number of network players can be 2 to 6 people. The full game requires membership of PlayStation®Plus for online multiplayer game access. Minimum 5 GB space is required. The DUALSHOCK®4 Vibration Function is required. HDTV screen resolution: 720p, 1080i, and 1080p. A PlayStation®Move navigation controller or a wireless controller is required for motion control features. PlayStation®VR and PlayStation®Camera are required to play this product. The game ranges from 90 to 120FPS.

The game "Robots Rescue" is played by one player. The DUALSHOCK®4 Vibration Function is required. HDTV screen resolution: 720p, 1080i, and 1080p. PlayStation®Move motion controller and PlayStation®Eye camera are optional. PlayStation®VR and PlayStation®Camera are required to play this product. The game ranges from 90FPS to 120FPS.

The game "Driveclub VR" is played by one player. The number of network players can be 2 to 8 people. The full game requires membership of PlayStation®Plus for online multiplayer game access. The DUALSHOCK®4 Vibration Function is required. HDTV screen resolution: 720p, 1080i, and 1080p. PlayStation®VR and PlayStation®Camera are required to play this product. The game ranges from 90FPS to 120FPS.

The game "Until Dawn" is played by one player. The DUALSHOCK®4 Vibration Function is required. HDTV screen resolution: 720p, 1080i, and 1080p. PlayStation®Move navigation controller and PlayStation®Eye camera are optional. PlayStation®VR and PlayStation®Camera are required to play this product. The game ranges from 90FPS to 120FPS.

The study was addressed in the context of the uses and effects approach. The uses and effects approach originated from the combination of uses and gratifications and the effect approach and attaches importance to revealing the analogies rather than the differences. In the model suggested by Sven Windahl, emphasis is placed on the quantity of the mass communication content consumed and on how it is consumed (Tekinalp and Uzun, 2009: 119; Uzun, 2013: 97). This model is acknowledged to be important in terms of its contribution to making predictions about the consequences of consumption.

Research

Our research aims to reveal whether the FPS change has any effect on users in the use of virtual reality headsets in the context of the uses and effects approach and, if yes, what kinds of effects it has. Within this scope, user experience made up of four different games with various levels of FPS changes in the virtual reality environment was performed through the conformity sampling of 50 people; the performances of the users during the game (when playing while standing) were observed; and interviews were made when the game was over in order to obtain user experiences as well as user feedback and views. Before the research, it had been determined which games the users would play and in what order as well as in which parts of the games attention would be paid to users' physical and verbal reactions (action accelerates or decelerates in certain parts of the games within the scope of the four games). During the observation, how the users reacted was particularly observed at certain points in the four games and these observations were recorded. To determine which parts of the games the researchers were going to pay attention to during the observation, they also experienced the four games. The FPS values of the four different games range from 90 to 120 in the game; and some of the four games address a calmer and slower style of playing, whereas some of them have a faster and more dynamic style of playing. By theme, the most FPS changes take place in Until Dawn, followed by Driveclub and Robots Rescue, respectively. The slowest and user-dependent FPS change takes place in Eagle Flight among the four games. In this sense, FPS was not further quantified and the reactions in the parts where the games accelerated and decelerated in the context of the FPS values shared by PlayStation were particularly watched.

In Game 1, namely Eagle Flight, the user only used the virtual reality headset and headphones but did not use any other tool. Game 1 is a type of action game and addresses people aged 7 years and over. In the First-Person Shooter-style game, the user tours above the city and its streets from the viewpoint of an eagle – the character in the game – by using head movements. While touring the city, he/she should find the eagle's nest, i.e. see the stimulus, or maneuver in various places of the city by using head movements during the tour. In this way, he/she is expected to experience and observe various figures created within the scope of the game. It was noted that all users played Game 1 for five minutes at the most.

In Game 2, namely Robots Rescue, the user used the console tool, along with the virtual reality headset and headphones. Game 2 is a type of action game and addresses people aged 3 years and over. In the role-playing-style game, the user tries to rescue the other robots that resemble it by moving a main character robot within the scope of the game on the island (with various actions such as by making it walk, jump, and walk on a rope), and while trying to collect the coins he/she meanwhile encounters, he/she tries to get a certain point or score and complete the game section within the scope of the time by escaping from monster robots, by beating them, and by blowing them up. It was noted whether the users were able to complete the section in Robots Rescue, and the duration of the game varied according to the performances of the users.

In Game 3, namely Driveclub, the user used the console tool, along with the virtual reality headset and headphones. Game 3 is a type of action game and addresses people aged 3 years and over. In the First-Person Shooter-style game, the user tries to complete the three rounds as the first in the shortest period of time by racing against the other race cars on the track defined within the scope of the game. While those who complete the three rounds in the shortest period of time within this scope get the highest point and score, the ranking is shaped according to this evaluation. It was noted whether the users were able to complete the section in the game, and the duration of the game varied according to the performances of the users.

In Game 4, namely Until Dawn, the user used the motion control stick, along with the virtual reality headset and headphones. Game 4 is a type of horror game and addresses people aged 18 years and over. In the First-Person Shooter-style game, the user should kill the zombies and shoot various stimuli like blue stars by using motion control sticks while proceeding in the tunnel in the game setting and complete the section by collecting points in a certain period of time in this way. Within this scope, the user should complete the game in a short period of time before he/she is damaged or killed by the zombies in Game 4. It was noted whether the users were able to complete the section in the game and the duration of the game varied according to the performances of the users.

The users were asked three questions after the experience:

1. Which game among the four games did you enjoy the most?
2. Which game among the four games did you enjoy the least or tensed you up the most?
3. Did you feel any negative effect during and after the game?

Enjoying or not enjoying a game, feeling tense during or after a game and giving physical and verbal reactions are related to whether a user can perform the missions in the game and to his/her getting of a score accordingly. In the games played by wearing a virtual reality headset, however, getting a good score is related to the ability to see the targets within the scope of the game clearly, perceiving them well, and the ability to shoot the targets or fulfill the missions accordingly. This is connected with the synchronous functioning of users' visual and sensory systems. While users with good visual and sensory perception systems complete the games easily without reacting to the games, the users who cannot see well or perceive well express this with various reactions and fail to get a good score. Within this scope, it is explicit that the FPS change in a game (i.e., seeing or failing to see the game image clearly or the sudden increase or drop, i.e. change, in FPS in certain parts) is related to the reactions of users in and after the game.

Within this scope, the research hypotheses are as follows:

H1: In the context of the uses and effects approach, the FPS change in the game has an effect on users in the games played by wearing a virtual reality headset.
H2: In the context of the uses and effects approach, the FPS change in the game causes users to give physical reactions in the games played by wearing a virtual reality headset.
H3: In the context of the uses and effects approach, the FPS change in the game causes users to give verbal reactions in the games played by wearing a virtual reality headset.
H4: In the context of the uses and effects approach, the stronger perception of the FPS change leads to physical reactions the most in the different games which are played by wearing a virtual reality headset and which the users state that they have enjoyed the most.
H5: In the context of the uses and effects approach, the stronger perception of the FPS change leads to physical reactions the most in the different games which are played by wearing a virtual reality headset and in which the users state that they have felt tense the most.
H6: In the context of the uses and effects approach, users' enjoyment of different games correlates with the physical reactions resulting from the FPS change.
H7: In the context of the uses and effects approach, the fact that the users state that they have felt tense in different games does not correlate with the physical reactions resulting from the FPS change.
H8: In the context of the uses and effects approach, the stronger perception of the FPS change leads to verbal reactions the most in the different games which are played by wearing a virtual reality headset and which the users state that they have enjoyed.
H9: In the context of the uses and effects approach, users' enjoyment of different games does not correlate with the verbal reactions resulting from the FPS change.
H10: In the context of the uses and effects approach, the stronger perception of the FPS change leads to verbal reactions the most in the different games which are played by wearing a virtual reality headset and in which the users state that they have felt tense.

H11: In the context of the uses and effects approach, the fact that the users state that they have felt tense in different games correlates with the verbal reactions resulting from the FPS change.
H12: In the context of the uses and effects approach, the FPS change in the game has negative effects on users in virtual reality games.

It was observed by the researchers that the 50 users gave physical and verbal reactions in various ways and in gradually increasing categorization within the scope of four different games and expressed negative effects after use. The observation data determined within the scope of the research were digitized and analyzed by means of the SPSS program. Accordingly, the distributions of frequencies of the physical and verbal reactions and expression of negative effects by the users within the scope of the four games and the median calculations for the physical and verbal reactions by game are as follows:

It was observed whether the users gave physical reactions in Game 1. Accordingly, it was observed that of them, 52 % did not give any physical reaction, 8 % gave minor physical reactions like moving their head rightwards and leftwards, again 8 % gave moderate physical reactions, and 32 % gave a high level of reactions such as being startled and bending the head when hitting – which were above the moderate level – while playing Game 1. It was observed whether the users gave verbal reactions in Game 1. Accordingly, it was seen that the users gave various levels of verbal reactions from muttering to themselves – the lowest way of talking – to screaming. It was observed that 34 % of the users did not give any verbal reaction at all, that 12 % of them muttered to themselves while playing the game, that 18 % of them talked to themselves or asked short questions to the observers during the game, that 18 % of them talked clearly, that 28 % of them gave slightly more verbal reactions than that in the previous category, and that 8 % of them gave the highest reaction and screamed within the scope of Game 1.

It was observed whether the users gave physical reactions in Game 2. Accordingly, it was observed that of them, 28 % did not give any physical reaction, 20 % gave minor physical reactions like moving their head rightwards and leftwards, again 24 % gave moderate physical reactions, and 28 % gave reactions at an above moderate, i.e. high level while playing Game 2. It was observed whether the users gave verbal reactions in Game 2. Accordingly, it was seen that the users gave various levels of verbal reactions from muttering to themselves – the lowest way of talking – to screaming. It was observed that 24 % of the users did not give any verbal reaction at all, that 22 % of them muttered to themselves while playing the game, that 28 % of them talked to themselves or asked short questions to the observers during the game, that 18 % of them continually talked clearly, that 4 % of them talked or gave verbal reactions more than that in the previous category group, and that 4 % of them gave the highest reaction and screamed or gave sudden verbal reactions loudly within the scope of Game 2.

It was observed whether the users gave physical reactions in Game 3. Accordingly, it was observed that of them, 32 % did not give any physical reaction, 16 % gave minor physical reactions such as slightly leaning or bending to the right and to the left at the bends, again 30 % gave moderate physical reactions, and 18 % gave physical reactions at a high level and were startled as the car crashed or bent rightwards and leftwards at the bends more exaggeratedly while playing Game 3. In addition, 4 % of the users gave the highest level of physical reaction for such reasons as nausea or dizziness during the car race and stated that they wanted to quit the game and it was observed that they stopped playing the game. It was observed whether the users gave verbal reactions in Game 3. Accordingly, it was seen that the users gave various levels of verbal reactions from muttering to themselves – the lowest way of talking – to screaming. It was observed that 48 % of the users did not give any verbal reaction, that 12 % of them muttered to themselves while playing the game, that 16 % of them talked to themselves or asked short questions to the observers during the game, that 18 % of them talked or gave verbal reactions more than that in the previous category group, and that 6 % of them gave the highest reaction and screamed or gave sudden verbal reactions loudly within the scope of Game 3.

It was observed whether the users gave physical reactions in Game 4. Accordingly, it was observed that of them, 12 % did not give any physical reaction, 24 % gave minor physical reactions such as withdrawing, being startled, slightly leaning to the right and to the left, and slightly bending their head, again 32 % gave moderate physical reactions, and 32 % gave physical reactions at a high level while playing Game 4. It was observed whether the users gave verbal reactions in Game 4. Accordingly, it was seen that the users gave various levels of verbal reactions from muttering to themselves – the lowest way of talking – to screaming. It was observed that 22 % of the users did not give any verbal reaction, that 12 % of them muttered to themselves while playing the game, that 32 % of them talked to themselves or asked short questions to the observers during the game, that 14 % of them talked or gave verbal reactions more than that in the previous category group, and that 20 % of them gave the highest reaction and screamed or gave sudden verbal reactions loudly within the scope of Game 4.

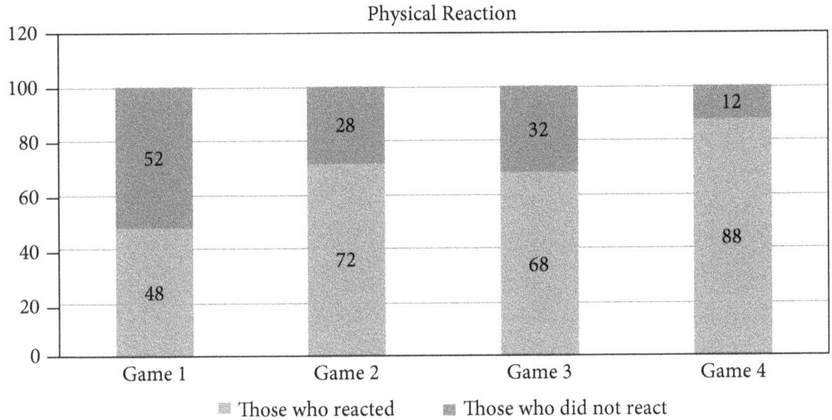

Graph 1: The Graph of the Physical Reactions by the Users During the Four Games.

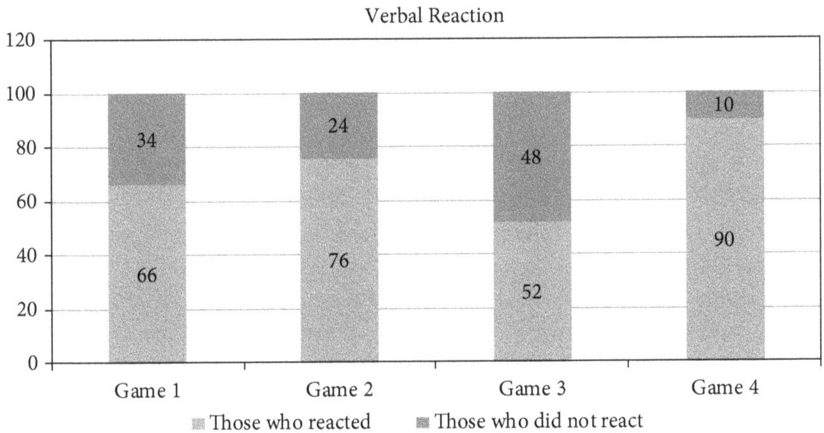

Graph 2: The Graph of Verbal Reactions by the Users During the Four Games.

As seen in Graphs 1 and 2, the physical and verbal reactions by the users gradually multiplied from Game 1 (from left) to the end of Game 4 (to right). In Game 4, namely Until Dawn, the change in FPS, i.e. its acceleration and deceleration alternately (for instance, the player's trying to shoot the targets while traveling in a cart, then the deceleration of the cart, and then its reacceleration), upon the use of horror elements ensures that both physical

Tab. 1: The Table of Physical Reactions in the Games According to the Most Enjoyed Game

	Game 1 physical reaction	Game 2 physical reaction	Game 3 physical reaction	Game 4 physical reaction
Of those stating that they enjoyed Eagle Flight the most				
Valid	8	8	8	8
Missing Value	0	0	0	0
Median	**3.50**	3.00	3.00	**3.50**
Of those stating that they enjoyed Robots Rescue the most				
Valid	16	16	16	16
Missing Value	0	0	0	0
Median	1.00	2.50	2.00	**4.50**
Of those stating that they enjoyed Driveclub the most				
Valid	7	7	7	7
Missing Value	0	0	0	0
Median	1.00	2.00	**3.00**	**3.00**
Of those stating that they enjoyed Until Dawn the most				
Valid	19	19	19	19
Missing Value	0	0	0	0
Median	1.00	2.00	**3.00**	**3.00**

and verbal reactions are at the highest level. The physical and verbal reactions categorically increased from the low level to stopping playing the game – the highest level – among the users. Only in Game 1, the rates of physical reactions were determined as 48 % for those who reacted and 52 % for those who did not react. However, the interaction of the user in the game is important in this game. That is, whether he/she gives a physical reaction depending on the FPS change is connected with the interaction of the user in the game. Accordingly, some players were observed to have chosen a calmer style of playing. Even despite this, the percentage of physical reactions observed for the game is high.

According to the above-mentioned findings, the hypothesis **"In the context of the uses and effects approach, the FPS change in the game has an effect on users in the games played by wearing a virtual reality headset."** (Hypothesis 1) was accepted. Depending on the acceptance of Hypothesis 1, the hypotheses **"In the context of the uses and effects approach, the FPS change in the game causes users to give physical reactions in the games played by wearing a virtual reality headset."** (Hypothesis 2) and **"In the context of the uses and effects approach, the FPS change in the game causes users to give verbal reactions in the games played by wearing a virtual reality headset."** (Hypothesis 3) were accepted.

Tab. 2: The Table of Physical Reactions in the Games According to the Game in which tension was felt the most

	Game 1 physical reaction	Game 2 physical reaction	Game 3 physical reaction	Game 4 physical reaction
Of those stating that they had been tensed up in Eagle Flight the most				
Valid	5	5	5	5
Missing Value	0	0	0	0
Median	1.00	2.00	2.00	**3.00**
Of those stating that they had been tensed up in Robots Rescue the most				
Valid	2	2	2	2
Missing Value	0	0	0	0
Median	**2.50**	1.00	1.00	1.50
Of those stating that they had been tensed up in Driveclub the most				
Valid	5	5	5	5
Missing Value	0	0	0	0
Median	1.00	2.00	4.00	**5.00**
Of those stating that they had been tensed up in Until Dawn the most				
Valid	38	38	38	38
Missing Value	0	0	0	0
Median	2.00	3.00	3.00	**4.00**

When the table of the physical reactions given in the games according to the games which the users stated that they had enjoyed the most is considered, it is seen that physical reactions were given in Until Dawn – Game 4 – the most. It is seen that all the users, who enjoyed the four different games, gave physical reactions in Game 4 the most (See Tab. 1, the downwards arrow). When the table of the physical reactions given in the games according to the different games in which tension was felt the most is considered, it is seen that Game 4 is at the highest level in three of the four games (See Tab. 2, the downwards arrow).

According to the above-mentioned findings, the hypothesis **"In the context of the uses and effects approach, the stronger perception of the FPS change leads to physical reactions the most in the different games which are played by wearing a virtual reality headset and which the users state that they have enjoyed the most."** (Hypothesis 4) was accepted. Again, the hypothesis **"In the context of the uses and effects approach, the stronger perception of the FPS change leads to physical reactions the most in the different games which are played by wearing a virtual reality headset and in which the users state that they have felt tense the most."** (Hypothesis 5) was accepted.

The physical reactions the users gave in different games according to the games which they stated that they had enjoyed the most, indicated with a cross-wise arrow, can be seen in Tab. 1. It is seen that 3/4 of the physical reactions of the users who stated that they had enjoyed different games were related to the game enjoyed. It is seen that only the users who stated that they had enjoyed Robots Rescue gave physical reactions (4.50) in Game 4 the most (See Tab. 1, the crosswise arrow). Hence, it is seen both that the users who stated that they had enjoyed different games the most gave physical reactions in the game with the most FPS changes and that the users who stated that they had enjoyed different games had high physical reaction values in these games.

According to the above-mentioned findings, the hypothesis **"In the context of the uses and effects approach, users' enjoyment of different games correlates with the physical reactions resulting from the FPS change."** (Hypothesis 6) was accepted.

The physical reactions the users gave in different games according to the games in which they stated that they had felt tense the most, indicated with a crosswise arrow, can be seen in Tab. 2. It is seen that the physical reactions of the users who stated that they had felt tense in different games were at the highest level in 2/4 of them (1.00, 1.00, 4.00, and 4.00, respectively) (See Tab. 2, the crosswise arrow).

According to the above-mentioned findings, the hypothesis **"In the context of the uses and effects approach, the fact that users state that they have felt tense in different games does not correlate with the physical reactions resulting from the FPS change."** (Hypothesis 7) was accepted.

When the table of the verbal reactions the users gave in the games according to the different games which they stated that they had enjoyed the most is considered (See Tab. 3), it is seen that they gave verbal reactions in Eagle Flight (Game 1) the most (3.50). It is seen that among the four different games enjoyed the most, the verbal reactions given within the scope of Game 1 the most were at the highest level in three of the four games (See Tab. 3, downwards, the highest 3.50, 3.00, 1.00, 3.00). The FPS change in Game 1 remains slower than that of Game 4; however, it is seen that verbal reactions were given in Game 1 the most. In Eagle Flight, the users were asked to tour the streets of the city and above the city. Since the users did not encounter any mission or target while touring in comparison with the other games, they felt it necessary to ask the researchers questions or talked to themselves. As what the users should do was slightly more uncertain in this game as compared with the other games; their comprehension of the game remained low; the users asked the researchers questions; and they demanded help from outside regarding what they should do within the scope of the game. Game 1 is a game in which the user should be directed. Thus, it is seen that the verbal reactions given within the scope of Game 1 were more than that in

Tab. 3: The Table of Verbal Reactions in the Games According to the Most Enjoyed Game

		Game 1 verbal reaction	Game 2 verbal reaction	Game 3 verbal reaction	Game 4 verbal reaction
Of those stating that they enjoyed Eagle Flight the most					
	Valid	8	8	8	8
	Missing Value	0	0	0	0
Median		**3.50**	**3.50**	3.00	**3.00**
Of those stating that they enjoyed Robots Rescue the most					
	Valid	16	16	16	16
	Missing Value	0	0	0	0
Median		**3.00**	2.00	2.00	2.50
Of those stating that they enjoyed Driveclub the most					
	Valid	7	7	7	7
	Missing Value	0	0	0	0
Median		1.00	2.00	1.00	**3.00**
Of those stating that they enjoyed Until Dawn the most					
	Valid	19	19	19	19
	Missing Value	0	0	0	0
Median		**3.00**	**3.00**	1.00	**3.00**

Until Dawn with a stronger FPS change. In other words, the verbal reactions (3.00) in Until Dawn with the strongest FPS change remained lower than that in Eagle Flight (3.50). Within this scope, it might be stated that users' giving of verbal reactions is in a sense related to their comprehension of the game.

According to the above-mentioned findings, the hypothesis **"In the context of the uses and effects approach, the stronger perception of the FPS change leads to verbal reactions the most in the different games which are played by wearing a virtual reality headset and which the users state that they have enjoyed."** (Hypothesis 8) was rejected.

Again, the verbal reactions the users gave in different games according to the games which they stated that they had enjoyed the most, indicated with a crosswise arrow, can be seen in Tab. 3. The correlation between 2/4 of the verbal reactions of the users who stated that they had enjoyed different games and the game enjoyed also confirms why Hypothesis 8 was rejected.

Thus, according to the above-mentioned findings, the hypothesis **"In the context of the uses and effects approach, users' enjoyment of different games does not correlate with the verbal reactions resulting from the FPS change."** (Hypothesis 9) was accepted.

Tab. 4: The Table of Verbal Reactions in the Games According to the Game in which Tension was felt the most

	Game 1 verbal reaction	Game 2 verbal reaction	Game 3 verbal reaction	Game 4 verbal reaction
Of those stating that Eagle Flight was the game in which tension was felt the most				
Valid	5	5	5	5
Missing Value	0	0	0	0
Median	**3.00**	2.00	1.00	**3.00**
Of those stating that Robots Rescue was the game in which tension was felt the most				
Valid	2	2	2	2
Missing Value	0	0	0	0
Median	2.00	**2.50**	1.50	1.00
Of those stating that Driveclub was the game in which tension was felt the most				
Valid	5	5	5	5
Missing Value	0	0	0	0
Median	3.00	3.00	2.00	**4.00**
Of those stating that Until Dawn was the game in which tension was felt the most				
Valid	38	38	38	38
Missing Value	0	0	0	0
Median	**3.00**	**3.00**	1.50	**3.00**

When the table of the verbal reactions given in the games according to the different games in which the users stated that they had felt tense the most is considered, it is seen that Until Dawn, Game 4, had the highest level of verbal reactions in three of the four games (See Tab. 4, downwards).

According to the above-mentioned findings, the hypothesis **"In the context of the uses and effects approach, the stronger perception of the FPS change in the different games which are played by wearing a virtual reality headset and in which the users state that they have felt tense leads to verbal reactions the most."** (Hypothesis 10) was accepted.

The verbal reactions the users gave in different games according to the games in which they stated that they had felt tense the most, indicated with a crosswise arrow, can be seen in Tab. 4. It is seen that the users who stated that they had felt tense in different games gave verbal reactions in the games in which they stated that they had felt tense the most.

According to the above-mentioned findings, the hypothesis **"In the context of the uses and effects approach, the fact that the users have felt tense in different games correlates with the verbal reactions resulting from the FPS change."** (Hypothesis 11) was accepted.

The negative effects expressed by the users after Game 1 were recorded. It was seen that the negative effects the users felt during the game were increasingly categorized. Accordingly, of the users, 24 % stated that there had been no negative effect, 10 % stated that they had felt first-level negative effects such as mild swaying and mild dizziness, 44 % stated that they had felt second-level negative effects, 16 % stated that they had felt such reactions as headache, dizziness, and swaying slightly more, and 6 % stated that they had felt use-induced negative effects at the highest level within the scope of Game 1. According to the findings, 24 % of the users did not feel any negative effect, whereas 76 % of them stated that they had felt negative effects in gradually increasing categorization depending on use in some way.

The negative effects expressed by the users after Game 2 were recorded. It was seen that the negative effects the users felt during the game were increasingly categorized. Accordingly, of the users, 10 % stated that there had been no negative effect, 6 % stated that they had felt first-level negative effects such as mild swaying and mild dizziness, 16 % stated that they had felt second-level negative effects, 52 % stated that they had felt such reactions as headache, dizziness, and swaying slightly more, and 16 % stated that they had felt use-induced negative effects at the highest level within the scope of Game 2. Accordingly, 90 % of the users in total stated that they had felt negative effects in gradually increasing categorization.

The negative effects expressed by the users after Game 3 were recorded. It was seen that the negative effects the users felt during the game were increasingly categorized. Accordingly, of the users, 10 % stated that there had been no negative effect, 8 % stated that they had felt first-level negative effects such as mild swaying and mild dizziness, 38 % stated that they had felt second-level negative effects, and 44 % stated that they had felt such reactions as headache, dizziness, and swaying slightly more within the scope of Game 3. Accordingly, 90 % of the users in total stated that they had felt negative effects in gradually increasing categorization.

The negative effects expressed by the users after Game 4 were recorded. It was seen that the negative effects the users felt during the game were increasingly categorized. Accordingly, of the users, 10 % stated that there had been no negative effect, 10 % stated that they had felt first-level negative effects such as mild swaying and mild dizziness, 28 % stated that they had felt second-level negative effects, 26 % stated that they had felt such reactions as headache, dizziness, and swaying slightly more and more severely than those in the other subcategories, and 26 % stated that they had felt use-induced negative effects at the highest level

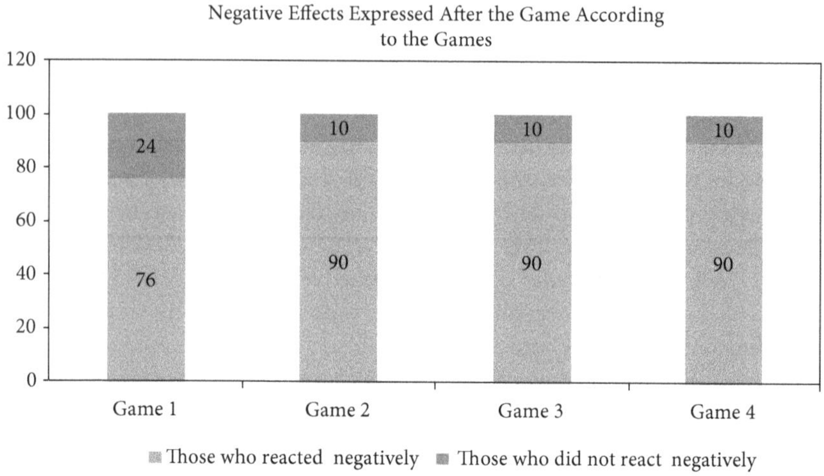

Graph 3: The Graph of the Use-Induced Negative Effects Expressed by the Users after the Four Games.

within the scope of Game 4. Accordingly, 90 % of the users in total stated that they had felt negative effects in gradually increasing categorization.

According to the above-mentioned findings, the hypothesis **"In the context of the uses and effects approach, the FPS change in the game has negative effects on users in virtual reality games."** (Hypothesis 12) was accepted as a result of the intensive perception of the FPS change in the games played by wearing all kinds of virtual reality headsets regardless of whether the users enjoyed the game or regardless of any game difference (The games played by the users are of such types of games. The one with the greatest value is the game called Until Dawn.).

Conclusion

Today virtual reality headsets are used within the scope of the game sector the most. Virtual reality headsets, which will perhaps become our new communication devices instead of mobile phones in the near future, have in a sense begun to shape the lifestyles of their users too. In this respect, we encounter not only the positive but also negative sides of virtual reality headsets, which have transformed the one-way communication of the conventional media into two-way interaction, depending on use. The negative symptoms resulting from the use of virtual reality headsets limit the possibility of the potential use of the communication technology in the future. Within this scope, the research performed intends to reveal whether the FPS change in the game has an effect on users depending on user experience in the context of the uses and effects approach and, if yes, what kinds of effects FPS has. In this respect, our research aims to examine the effects of the FPS change – the state of noise in the fundamental communication model which has been carried to the virtual reality environment – on users. No other FPS quantification was performed, and the FPS data shared by PlayStation were taken as the basis. In this context, it is known that the FPS value increases when the image in the game accelerates but decreases when it decelerates.

Within this scope and in the context of the uses and effects approach, the first and most important result of the research is that the FPS change in the game caused users to give physical and verbal reactions in the games played by wearing a virtual reality headset.

The second result is that in the context of the uses and effects approach, the stronger perception of the FPS change led to physical reactions the most in the different games which were played by wearing a virtual reality headset and which the users stated that they had enjoyed or in which they stated that they had felt tense. That is, physical reactions are given at the highest level in the games with intensive FPS changes and this is appreciated by users. Additionally, the low level of physical reactions by the users in the games in which they felt tense the most reveals that there is a linear relationship among user enjoyment, the FPS change, and physical reactions. That is, it is possible to state that intensive FPS changes are made consciously, in a way that will increase the physical reactions of users, and in order to provide user enjoyment. Besides, to attain users' enjoyment the most, the FPS change is organized to ensure physical reactions the most. In this sense, within the scope of the use of virtual reality headsets, the FPS change is used to enhance users' enjoyment.

In addition, the stronger perception of the FPS change did not lead to verbal reactions the most in the different games which were played by wearing a virtual reality headset and which the users stated that they had enjoyed, which demonstrates that the FPS change did not correlate with whether a verbal reaction was given. It is possible to think that in virtual reality, the FPS change is created to enable users to give physical, but not verbal, reactions the most and that users are enabled to get pleasure within this scope. In this respect, it is observed that the FPS change is organized to enable users to get pleasure from the game.

The third result is that naturally, the strong perception of the FPS change led to verbal reactions the most in the different games which were played by wearing a virtual reality headset and in which the users stated that they had felt tense. By theme, the verbal reactions of the players multiply in terrifying environments.

The fourth result within the scope of the research is that in the context of the uses and effects approach, the FPS change in the game had negative effects on the users in the virtual reality games. It was observed that the negative symptoms could reach increasing categorization from mild swaying and mild dizziness to quitting the game before being able to complete it. The FPS change used for an increase in the use of virtual reality headsets and so as to enhance the pleasure the users get from the environment leads to negative symptoms on users depending on the use of virtual reality headsets. This occurs as the greatest obstacle to the increase in the use of virtual reality headsets and to the development of the relevant industry.

To briefly summarize and interpret the four results, the strong FPS change increases immersion and hence enhances the sense of presence. While this increases the physical reactions of users, it also enables them to get pleasure from the game and enjoy it. In this sense, it is possible to state that the FPS change enhances users' enjoyment. Nevertheless, in this research, it turned out that the FPS change led to use-induced negative symptoms and multiplied these negative symptoms.

Bibliography

Adorno, T. W. (2012). Kültür Endüstrisi. İstanbul: İletişim Yayınları.

Barrett, J. (2004). Side Effects of Virtual Environments: A Review of the Literature. Australia: Department of Defence, Defence Science Technology Organisation Information Sciences Laboratory. Retrieved from https://pdfs.semanticscholar.org/ab1b/4153e44abb4c1a1fcac5f2aaee847d30ecf3.pdf on 12 March 2018.

Baudrillard, J. (2005). Simülakrlar ve Simülasyon. Ankara: Doğu Batı Yayınları.

Chayko, M. (2018). Süperbağ(lantı)lı: İnternet, Dijital Medya & Tekno-Sosyal Hayat. İstanbul: Der Yayınları.

Chen, C. H., Ho, C. H. & Lin, J. B. (2015). The Development of an Augmented Reality Game-Based Learning Environment. Procedia – Social and Behavioral Sciences, 174, 216–220.

Cobb, S., Nichols, S., Ramsey, A. & Wilson, J. R. (1999). Virtual Reality-Induced Symptoms and Effects (VRISE). Presence: Teleoperators and Virtual Environments, 8(2), 169–186.

Duh, H. B. L., Lin, J. J. W., Kenyon, R. V., Parker, D. E. & Furness, T.A. (2001). Effects of Field of View on Balance in an Immersive Environment. Proceedings of IEEE Virtual Reality. Yokohama, Japan.

Ellul, J. (2003). Teknoloji Toplumu. İstanbul: Bakış Yayınevi.

Foucault, M. (2003). İktidarın Gözü. İstanbul: Ayrıntı Yayınları.

Freeman, D., Reeve, S., Robinson, A., Ehlers, A., Clark, D., Spanlang, B. & Slater, M. (2017). Virtual Reality in the Assessment, Understanding, and Treatment of Mental Health Disorders. Psychological Medicine, 47, 2393–2400.

Hitchcock, L. A. (2013). Kuramlar ve Kuramcılar. İstanbul: İletişim Yayınları.

Innis, H. A. (2006). İmparatorluk ve İletişim Araçları. Ankara: Ütopya Yayınları.

iWazzuu. (2010, January 10). GoPro HD Hero 30fps vs. 60fps [Video File]. Retrieved from https://www.youtube.com/watch?v=-nU2_ERC_oE on 2 May 2018.

Karadağ, G. H. (2017). What Does Periscope Offer to Professional and Citizen Reporters? A Sample Study from Turkey. The Turkish Online Journal of Design, Art and Communication–TOJDAC, 7(4), 709–727.

King, B. (2016). Augmented. İstanbul: MediaCat.

Kolasinski, E. M. (1995). Simulator Sickness in Virtual Environments. Technical Report (No. ARI-TR-1027). U.S. Army Research Institute for the Behavioral and Social Sciences, Virginia. Retrieved from https://www.resonant.org/text/simulator_sickness_report.html on 26 July 2017.

Lin, J. J. W. & Parker D. E. (2007). User Experience Modeling and Enhancement for Virtual Environments That Employ Wide-Field Displays. In V. G. Duff y (Ed.), Digital Human Modeling. Proceedings of the 1st international Conference on Digital Human Modeling (pp. 423–433). Beijing, China.

Lin, J. J. W., Duh, H. B. L., Parker, D. E., Abi-Rached, H. & Furness, T. A. (2002). Effects of Field of View on Presence, Enjoyment, Memory, and Simulator Sickness in a Virtual Environment. In B. Loftin, J. X. Chen, S. Rizzo, M. Goebel, and M. Hirose (Eds.) Conference Proceedings of IEEE Virtual Reality 2002 (pp. 164–171). Orlando, FLorida, USA.

Manovich, L. (2001). The Language of New Media. Cambridge: The MIT Press.

McCauley, M. E. & Sharkey, T. J. (1992). Cybersickness: Perception of Self-Motion in Virtual Environments. Presence: Teleoperators & Virtual Environments, 1(3), 311–318.

McLuhan, M. (2001). Global Köy. İstanbul: Scala Yayıncılık.

Motion Compensated Video Deinterlacing and Framerate Conversion. (n.d.). Retrieved from http://www.ifp.illinois.edu/~yuhuang/MEMCI.html on 10 May 2018.

Nichols, S., Haldane, C. & Wilson, J. R. (2000a). Measurement of Presence and Its Consequences in Virtual Environments. International Journal of Human-Computer Studies, 52(3), 471–491.

Nichols, S., Ramsey, A. D., Cobb, S., Neale, H., D'Cruz, M. & Wilson, J. R. (2000b). Incidence of Virtual Reality Symptoms and Effects (VRISE) in

Desktop and Projection Screen Displays. Sudbury Norwich: HSE Books. Retrieved from http://www.hse.gov.uk/research/crr_pdf/2000/crr00274.pdf on 12 April 2018.

Ong, W. J. (1995). Sözlü ve Yazılı Kültür. İstanbul: Metis Yayınları.

Oppenheim, C. (1993). Virtual Reality and the Virtual Library. Information Services and Use, 13(3), 215–227.

Orwell, G. (2016). 1984. İstanbul: Can Yayınları.

Oskay, Ü. (1993). XIX. Yüzyıldan Günümüze Kitle İletişiminin Kültürel İşlevleri. İstanbul: Der Yayınları.

Ottosson, S. (2002). Virtual Reality in the Product Development Process. Journal of Engineering Design, 13, 159–172.

Pausch, R., Crea, T. & Conway, M. (1992). A Literature Survey for Virtual Environments: Military Flight Simulator Visual Systems and Simulator Sickness. Presence, 1(3), 344–363. Retrieved from http://www.cs.cmu.edu/~stage3/publications/93/journals/PRESENCE/militaryFlight/paper.html on 26 July 2017.

Pimentel, K. & Teixeira, K. (1993). Virtual Reality, Through the Looking Glass. New York: Windcrest/McGraw Hill.

PlayStation.Store. (2015). WRC 5 FIA World Rally Championship. Retrieved from https://store.playstation.com/tr-tr/product/EP4008-PCSB00762_00-WRC5000000000000 on 26 May 2018.

Sharples, S., Cobb, S., Moody, A. & Wilson, J. R. (2008). Virtual Reality Induced Symptoms and Effects (VRISE): Comparison of Head Mounted Display (HMD). Desktop and Projection Display Systems. Displays, 29(2), 58–69.

Sherman, W. R. & Craig, A. B. (2003). Understanding Virtual Reality. USA: Elsevier Science.

Sherman, W. R., Craig A. B. & Will, J. D. (2009). Developing Virtual Reality Application, Foundation of Effective Design. China: Morgan Kaufmann Publication.

So, R. H. Y., Ho, A. T. K. & Lo, W. T. (2001). A Metric to Quantify Virtual Scene Movement for the Study of Cybersickness: Definition, Implementation, and Verification. Presence: Teleoperators & Virtual Environments, 10(2), 193–215.

Staff. (2014, Jun 2). Frames Per Second: 5 Simple Tips to Boost Your FPS [Blog post]. Retrieved fromhttp://blog.logicalincrements.com/2014/06/frames-per-second-5-simple-tips-to-boost-your-fps/ on 11 May 2018.

Stanney, K. ve Salvendy, G. (1998). Aftereffects and Sense of Presence in Virtual Environments: Formulation of a Research and Development Agenda. International Journal of Human-Computer Interaction, 10(2), 135–187.

Tekinalp, Ş. & Uzun, R. (2009). İletişim Araştırmaları ve Kuramları. İstanbul: Beta Basım.

Usoh, M., Catena, E., Arman, S. & Slater, M. (2000). Using Presence Questionnaires in Reality. Presence: Teleoperators and Virtual Environment, 9(5), 497–503.

Uzun, R. (2013). İzleyici Merkezli Yaklaşımlar. In E. Yüksel (Ed.), İletişim Kuramları (pp. 84–105). Eskişehir: T.C. Anadolu Üniversitesi Yayınları.

Valmaggia, L.R., Latif, L., Kempton, M. J. & Rus-Calafell, M. (2016). Virtual Reality in the Psychological Treatment for Mental Health Problems. A Systematic Review of Recent Evidence. Psychiatry Research, 236, 189–195.

Van Dijk, J. (2016). Ağ Toplumu. İstanbul: Kafka Yayınevi.

Virilio, P. (2003). Enformasyon Bombası. İstanbul: Metis Yayınları.

What is an action camera? (2018). Noticery Review. Retrieved from http://noticery.com/what-is-an-action-camera/ on 4 January 2019.

Welch, R. B., Blackmon, T. T., Liu, A., Mellers, B. A. & Stark, L. W. (1996). The Effects of Pictorial Realism, Delay of Visual Feedback, and Observer Interactivity on the Subjective Sense of Presence. Presence: Teleoperators and Virtual Environments, 5(3), 263–273.

Yaylagül, L. (2016). Kitle İletişim Kuramları. Ankara: Dipnot Yayınları.

Yengin, D. (2014). Yeni Medya ve Dokunmatik Toplum. İstanbul: Derin Yayınları.

Yengin, D. & Bayrak, T. (2018). Sanal Gerçeklik VR. İstanbul: Der Yayınları.

List of Figures

Deniz Yengin and Berkan Bayındır
Digitally Connected and/or Addicted

Didem Ataman Yengin
Digital Game Addiction

Tamer Bayrak and And Algül
Effects of Frame Rate in Virtual Reality

List of Tables

Index

About the Writers

AND ALGÜL

And Algül, born in 1973, graduated from Bilkent University, took his master's degree from Marmara University, and completed his PhD at Yeditepe University. He, working as a lecturer at Istanbul Aydin University, Faculty of Communication, Department of Visual Communication Design Studies, conducts studies about Virtual Reality, Informatics Society, Surveillance Society, Technological Determinism, Social Media, New Media, Interaction, Culture, Society, Design, Digital Games and Communication Tools.

AYTEN ÖVÜR

Ayten Övür, born in 1974, Fatsa, graduated from Marmara University, Department of Journalism. Övür, who started her career as a journalist in Marmara University News Agency (MİHA), worked as a reporter in Nokta Magazines. She studied at University of California for television journalism and worked as a photojournalist in *The Resident Newspaper*, in New York. Övür, working as an internet editor in tv8, has completed her master and doctorate degrees in Communication Sciences, at the Department of Radio and Television at Marmara University. Plus, she worked as an editor of "with Mithat Bereket +1" program. She worked as an editor of foreign news in Dogan News Agency after she had taken a Spanish education in Cuba and Peru. Övür, who is Assistant Manager of IAU New Media Application and Research Center, still works as a doctor lecturer at Istanbul Aydin University.

BERKAN BAYINDIR

Berkan Bayındır, born in 1975, Ankara, graduated from Hacettepe University, Faculty of Economics and Administrative Sciences, Department of Tourism and Hotel Management. After that, he got his BA degree in English Language Teaching at the Faculty of Educational Sciences at Ondokuz Mayis University. Mr. Bayındır, working as an English teacher at the Ministry of Education, completed his master's degree at the Beykent University, Institute of Social Sciences, Department of Business Administration, Education Management and Control with the thesis titled "Home Visit in School-Family Communication". He currently works as English Teacher at an Anatolian High School affiliated to the Ministry of Education, and continues his PhD at Istanbul Aydin University, Department of Public Relations and Publicity.

DENİZ YENGİN

Deniz Yengin, born in 1978, Istanbul, graduated from Istanbul Bilgi University, Faculty of Economics and Administrative Sciences, Department of Economics as a bachelor. He completed his master's degree in Istanbul Kültür University Institute of Social Sciences Communication Design Program. He took his doctorate from Marmara University Institute of Social Sciences, Department of Informatics. He is lecturer at IAU Faculty of Communication, Head of the Department of New Media and Communication and director of IAU New Media Practice and Research Center; he studies on Scientific Research Methods, Virtual Reality, Big Data, Internet of Things, Informatics Society, Surveillance Society, Technological Determinism, Touch Society, Social Media, New Media, Digital Games and Media.

DİDEM ATAMAN YENGİN

Didem Ataman Yengin, born in 1979, Istanbul, completed her undergraduate education in Istanbul Bilgi University and Eskişehir Anadolu University, Department of Management. She completed her master's degree in Istanbul Kültür University Institute of Social Sciences Communication Arts Program and her thesis subject was "Advertorials as a Medium of Consumption Culture and Anthropomorphism (object people or humanoids). Yengin, who completed her doctorate program in Istanbul Aydın University Institute of Social Sciences, Department of Public Relations and Publicity, gives lectures on master degree and undergraduate lessons about Digital Addiction, Social Media, Advertising and Sponsorship.

GÖKMEN H. KARADAĞ

Gökmen H. Karadağ, born in 1970, in Erzincan, received his bachelor's degree from Boğaziçi University, Industrial Engineering Department. After a short period of engineering career, he shifted to media and communication industry. He worked as writer, reporter, editor, producer and anchor during his TV career. He got his master's and doctorate degrees from Institute of Social Sciences, Marmara University, focusing on TV News Programming and European Communication Policies, respectively. He is currently working as Assistant Professor at İstanbul Aydın University, Department of New Media and Communication. He is also a member of the research team of Virtual Reality Laboratory at İstanbul Aydın University.

NUR EMİNE KOÇ

Nur Emine Koç, born in 1980, got her B.A. and M.A. degree in English Language and Literature Department; after that, she studied Communication Sciences for PhD at Maltepe University in 2016. Her doctoral thesis associating these two branches of science is called "An Example of Reality Show Programs on Television as a part of Consumer Society: "Evim Şahane" Program. She has translated the Entrepreneurship book, being taught at Istanbul Aydın University for six years, into English. In her international and national articles, she has also worked in the context of literature branches and radio, television and cinema. Koç is currently the Vice Principal for Vocational School of Foreign Languages, the Head of English Translation and Interpreting and Applied English and Translation Program, and she has been working as Coordinator of the Foreign Language Education at Istanbul Aydın University. She is a 16-year educator and has been working at Istanbul Aydın University since 2011.

ÖZGE TOPÇU

Born in 1984 in Istanbul, Özge Topçu graduated from Faculty of Art and Design in the Department of Communication Arts. She completed her master's degree in Public Relations at the Faculty of Communication at Marmara University. She got her doctorate education in the Public Relations and Publicity Program of the Institute of Social Science at Istanbul Aydın University. Furthermore, Topçu studies on Corporate Identity, Digital Publishing, Technological Determinism and Communication.

TAMER BAYRAK

Tamer Bayrak was born in 1988 in Istanbul. He graduated from Faculty of Art and Design in the Department of Communication Design. He completed his master's degree in the Communication Design Program at the Institute of Social Sciences at Istanbul Kültür University. He has been continuing his doctorate education in the Public Relations and Publicity Program of the Institute of Social Science at Istanbul Aydın University. Bayrak, being a research assistant in the New Media and Communication Department at the Faculty of Communication at Istanbul Aydın University; studies on Virtual Reality, New Media, Digital Games, Technological Determinism, Research Methods and Communication.

www.ingramcontent.com/pod-product-compliance
Ingram Content Group UK Ltd.
Pitfield, Milton Keynes, MK11 3LW, UK
UKHW021847100926
8556IPUK00020B/1098

9 783631 805534